Table of Contents

Tell Me About Marfan Syndrome

How was Marfan Syndrome discovered?

Marfan syndrome was named after the French physician Antoine Marfan, who first described the disorder in 1896. Dr. Marfan encountered a young girl who exhibited several distinct physical characteristics and abnormalities. He noted her unusually long limbs, slender fingers, and loose joints, along with other manifestations such as a sunken chest and abnormal curvature of the spine.

Intrigued by this collection of symptoms, Dr. Marfan continued to study and document similar cases, ultimately publishing his findings in medical literature. His observations and subsequent research helped establish Marfan syndrome as a distinct medical condition.

Since then, further advancements have been made in understanding the genetic basis of Marfan syndrome. In the 1990s, scientists discovered that mutations in the FBN1 gene, which codes for the fibrillin-1 protein, are responsible for the majority of cases. Fibrillin-1 is a vital component of connective tissue, and alterations in this gene can disrupt the structural integrity of various body systems, leading to the characteristic features and complications seen in Marfan syndrome.

Through ongoing research and medical advancements, our understanding of Marfan syndrome has improved, allowing for better diagnosis, management, and treatment of individuals with the condition.

Marfan syndrome is a genetic disorder that affects the body's connective tissue. Connective tissue is a type of tissue that helps to hold the body together. It is found in the bones, muscles, blood vessels, and other organs.

What is Marfan Syndrome?

Marfan syndrome is caused by a mutation in the FBN1 gene. This gene is responsible for making a protein called fibrillin-1. Fibrillin-1 is a major component of connective tissue. When the FBN1 gene is mutated, it makes less fibrillin-1, or the fibrillin-1 that is made is not as strong. This can lead to problems with the development and function of connective tissue.

The symptoms of Marfan syndrome can vary from person to person. Some common symptoms include:

Tall and thin body build

Long, thin arms and legs

Elongated fingers and toes

Pectus carinatum (protruding chest) or pectus excavatum (sunken chest)

Scoliosis (curvature of the spine)

Loose joints

Myopia (nearsightedness)

Aortic aneurysm (enlargement of the aorta)

Mitral valve prolapse (a condition in which the mitral valve in the heart does not close properly)

Dislocation of the lens in the eye

Marfan syndrome is a serious condition that can lead to a number of health problems. The most serious complications of Marfan syndrome are related to the heart and blood vessels. An aortic aneurysm is a bulge in the aorta, the main artery that carries blood away from the heart. If the aortic aneurysm ruptures, it can be fatal. Mitral valve prolapse is a condition in which the mitral valve in the heart does not close properly. This can cause blood to leak back into the heart, which can lead to heart failure.

There is no cure for Marfan syndrome, but there are treatments that can help to manage the symptoms and prevent complications. Treatment for Marfan syndrome typically includes:

Regular checkups with a doctor to monitor for signs of complications

Medications to control high blood pressure and other risk factors for heart disease

Surgery to repair or replace an aortic aneurysm

Surgery to repair or replace a mitral valve

With early diagnosis and treatment, people with Marfan syndrome can live long and healthy lives.

Learn More about Marfan Syndrome from

'THE MARFAN FOUNDATION'

The Marfan Foundation

2500 Marcus Avenue

Port Washington, NY 11050

The Marfan Foundation

1901 W. Wellington Ave. Suite 300

Chicago, IL 60614

Tell me about Ehlers-Danlos syndrome

How was Ehlers-Danlos syndrome discovered?

Ehlers-Danlos syndrome (EDS) was first described in 1901 by Danish dermatologist Edvard Ehlers and French pediatrician Henri-Alexandre Danlos. They independently reported patients with a rare disorder characterized by hypermobility of the joints, stretchy skin, and easy bruising.

In the years since its discovery, EDS has been classified into several types, each with its own set of symptoms. The most common type of EDS is hypermobility type, which is characterized by loose joints and stretchy skin. Other types of EDS include classical EDS, vascular EDS, and kyphoscoliotic EDS.

EDS is a genetic disorder, which means that it is caused by changes in the DNA. The exact genes that cause EDS are still being studied, but scientists believe that there are at least 10 different genes that can be involved.

EDS is a lifelong condition, and there is no cure. However, there are treatments that can help to manage the symptoms and improve the quality of life for people with EDS. These treatments may include physical therapy, pain medication, and surgery.

With early diagnosis and treatment, people with EDS can live long and productive lives.

Here are some additional details about the different types of EDS:

Hypermobility type EDS: This is the most common type of EDS, and it is characterized by loose joints and stretchy skin. People with hypermobility type EDS may also experience pain, fatigue, and poor circulation.

Classical EDS: This type of EDS is characterized by loose joints, stretchy skin, and easy bruising. People with classical EDS may also experience heart problems, aortic aneurysms, and mitral valve prolapse.

Vascular EDS: This type of EDS is the most serious type of EDS, and it is characterized by loose joints, stretchy skin, and easy bruising. People with vascular EDS are at risk for life-threatening complications, such as aortic aneurysms and ruptures.

Kyphoscoliotic EDS: This type of EDS is characterized by loose joints, stretchy skin, and kyphoscoliosis (a curvature of the spine). People with kyphoscoliotic EDS may also experience scoliosis, breathing problems, and heart problems.

What is Ehlers-Danlos Syndrome?

Ehlers-Danlos syndrome (EDS) is a group of rare genetic disorders that affect the connective tissues in the body. Connective tissues provide support and structure to various organs, including the skin, joints, blood vessels, and organs. EDS is characterized by a defect in the production, processing, or structure of collagen, which is the main component of connective tissue.

There are several different types of EDS, each with its own set of symptoms and genetic causes. The most common types include:

Classical EDS (cEDS): This type is characterized by stretchy and fragile skin, joint hypermobility, and a tendency to develop scars and widened scars easily. It can also affect blood vessels and internal organs.

Hypermobility EDS (hEDS): Individuals with hEDS have joint hypermobility, which means their joints have a wider range of motion than usual. They may also experience chronic joint pain, loose and unstable joints, and skin that is soft and stretchy.

Vascular EDS (vEDS): This is the most severe and potentially life-threatening form of EDS. It affects the blood vessels, causing them to be fragile and prone to rupture. Individuals with vEDS may have thin, translucent skin, easily bruised skin, organ ruptures, and arterial dissections.

Other less common types of EDS include kyphoscoliotic EDS, arthrochalasia EDS, dermatosparaxis EDS, and more.

The symptoms of EDS can vary widely depending on the type and severity. Common symptoms include joint hypermobility, skin hyperextensibility, easy bruising, chronic pain, fragile blood vessels, gastrointestinal issues, and problems with healing and scarring. Some individuals may also experience complications such as joint dislocations, early-onset osteoarthritis, cardiac abnormalities, and organ prolapse.

EDS is typically diagnosed through a thorough clinical examination, medical history, and genetic testing. While there is no cure for EDS, treatment mainly focuses on managing symptoms and preventing complications. This may involve physical therapy, pain management strategies, bracing or splinting, surgery for specific issues, and regular monitoring of organ function in severe cases.

It's important for individuals with EDS to work closely with healthcare professionals, such as geneticists, rheumatologists, and physiotherapists, to develop a personalized management plan and ensure proper care and support.

Learn more about Ehlers-Danlos Syndrome from

'The Ehlers-Danlos Society'

The Ehlers-Danlos Society

447 Broadway, 2nd FL #670

New York, NY 10013

Satellite Office :

The Ehlers-Danlos Society

2nd Floor, 125 Old Gloucester Street

London, WC1N 3AX

United Kingdom

Tell Me About Cornelia de Lange Syndrome

How was Cornelia de Lange syndrome discovered?

Cornelia de Lange syndrome (CdLS) was first described in 1933 by Cornelia de Lange, a Dutch pediatrician. She described two unrelated girls with similar features, including:

Growth retardation

Intellectual disability

Microcephaly

Brachycephaly

Epicanthic folds

Low-set ears

Long eyelashes

Hirsutism

Webbing of the neck

Clinodactyly

Pectus excavatum

Heart defects

CdLS is a rare genetic disorder caused by mutations in one of several genes. The most common gene affected is NIPBL, which is located on chromosome 5. Mutations in NIPBL disrupt the development of cells during the embryo's early development, leading to the characteristic features of CdLS.

There is no cure for CdLS, but there are treatments available to help manage the symptoms. These treatments may include:

Growth hormone therapy

Speech therapy

Occupational therapy

Physical therapy

Special education

With appropriate care, people with CdLS can live long and fulfilling lives.

Here are some additional details about the discovery of CdLS:

The two girls that de Lange described were both born in Amsterdam, Netherlands.

The girls were not related, but they had very similar physical features.

De Lange named the syndrome after herself, and it has been known by that name ever since.

In the years since de Lange's discovery, much more has been learned about CdLS.

Researchers have identified the genes that cause CdLS, and they have developed treatments to help manage the symptoms.

Despite the challenges that people with CdLS face, they can live long and fulfilling lives.

What is Cornelia de Lange Syndrome?

Cornelia de Lange syndrome (CdLS), also known as Brachmann-de Lange syndrome, is a rare genetic disorder that affects multiple organ systems and leads to a wide range of physical, cognitive, and developmental challenges. CdLS is typically caused by mutations in genes related to the cohesin complex, a protein complex involved in regulating the structure and function of chromosomes.

The syndrome was first described by Dutch pediatrician Cornelia de Lange in 1933, and additional contributions were made by German physician Brachmann in the 1970s, hence the name Cornelia de Lange syndrome.

Some common features and characteristics of CdLS include:

Facial Features: Individuals with CdLS often have distinct facial characteristics, such as arched eyebrows, long eyelashes, thin upper lip, a small upturned nose, and small widely spaced teeth.

Growth and Development: CdLS can be associated with growth deficiency, resulting in short stature. Developmental delays are common, including cognitive impairments, speech and language delays, and motor coordination difficulties.

Limb Abnormalities: Limb abnormalities may include small hands and feet, partial fusion of the fingers or toes (syndactyly), and limited range of motion in the joints.

Gastrointestinal Issues: Many individuals with CdLS experience gastrointestinal problems, such as gastroesophageal reflux (GERD), feeding difficulties, and constipation.

Cardiac and Renal Anomalies: Structural heart defects and kidney abnormalities can occur in some individuals with CdLS.

Behavioral and Psychological Challenges: Individuals with CdLS may exhibit behavioral challenges, including self-injurious behaviors, hyperactivity, anxiety, and repetitive movements.

The severity of CdLS can vary widely among affected individuals. Some individuals may have mild to moderate features, while others may have more severe symptoms that significantly impact their daily lives.

Diagnosis of CdLS is typically based on clinical evaluation and recognition of characteristic features. Genetic testing can confirm the diagnosis by identifying mutations in genes associated with CdLS, such as NIPBL, SMC1A, or SMC3.

Management of CdLS involves a multidisciplinary approach, addressing the various medical, developmental, and behavioral aspects of the syndrome. Treatment may include early intervention programs, speech and occupational therapy, specialized educational support, feeding assistance, and addressing associated medical issues on an individual basis.

It's important for individuals with CdLS and their families to receive comprehensive medical care and support from healthcare professionals experienced in managing the syndrome to optimize their quality of life and well-being.

Find out more about Cornelia de Lange Syndrome at CdLS Foundation

Cornelia de Lange Syndrome Foundation

30 Tower Lane, Suite 400

Avon, CT 06001

(800) 753-2357

Tell Me About Rett Syndrome

How was Rett Syndrome discovered?

Rett syndrome was first described and discovered by Austrian physician Dr. Andreas Rett in 1966. Dr. Rett observed a group of girls with similar symptoms and developmental regression, and he published his findings in a medical journal, initially referring to the condition as "cerebroatrophic hyperammonemia."

Dr. Rett's work largely went unnoticed until the late 1980s when Swedish geneticist Dr. Bengt Hagberg rediscovered the syndrome independently. Dr. Hagberg named it "Rett syndrome" to honor Dr. Rett's original observation and contribution.

The rediscovery of Rett syndrome drew attention to the disorder, leading to increased research and awareness. Dr. Hagberg and his colleagues conducted further investigations into the condition, characterizing the clinical features and establishing it as a distinct clinical entity.

In the late 1990s, scientists made a significant breakthrough in understanding Rett syndrome by identifying mutations in the MECP2 gene as the primary cause. The MECP2 gene plays a crucial role in regulating gene expression and is critical for the normal development and function of the brain.

This discovery was a major milestone in understanding Rett syndrome and its genetic basis. Subsequent research has further expanded our knowledge of the syndrome, including its wide-ranging clinical spectrum, underlying genetic mutations, and potential treatment strategies.

Today, Rett syndrome is recognized as a rare genetic disorder primarily affecting girls. It is characterized by normal development in early infancy followed by a loss of acquired skills, motor difficulties, repetitive hand movements (such as hand-wringing), severe communication impairments, breathing abnormalities, and intellectual disability.

Continued research and advancements in understanding Rett syndrome have contributed to improved diagnosis, management, and support for individuals and families affected by this complex neurological disorder.

What is Rett Syndrome?

Rett syndrome is a rare genetic disorder that primarily affects girls. It is a neurodevelopmental disorder characterized by a period of normal development followed by a loss of acquired skills and a regression in motor, cognitive, and social abilities. The syndrome is named after Dr. Andreas Rett, the Austrian physician who first described it.

Here are some key features and characteristics of Rett syndrome:

Developmental Regression: Rett syndrome typically manifests between 6 and 18 months of age, when a period of developmental stagnation or regression occurs. Skills that were previously acquired, such as purposeful hand use, social engagement, and language development, start to deteriorate.

Loss of Motor Skills: Individuals with Rett syndrome experience a loss of purposeful hand movements and the development of stereotypical hand movements, such as hand-wringing, clapping, or tapping. Gross motor skills, such as walking, may also be affected, leading to gait abnormalities or a loss of mobility.

Communication Impairments: Rett syndrome often involves severe communication difficulties. Verbal language may be lost or significantly impaired, and nonverbal communication methods, such as eye contact, gestures, or vocalizations, may also be affected.

Cognitive Impairment: Intellectual disability is common in individuals with Rett syndrome. The severity of cognitive impairment can vary, ranging from mild to severe. Some individuals may have preserved social engagement and understanding despite significant cognitive challenges.

Breathing Abnormalities: Individuals with Rett syndrome may exhibit breathing abnormalities, including irregular breathing patterns, hyperventilation, breath-holding, or periods of apnea (temporary cessation of breathing).

Behavioral and Motor Issues: Rett syndrome can involve behavioral issues, including anxiety, social withdrawal, agitation, and autistic-like behaviors. Motor abnormalities such as muscle stiffness, poor coordination, and abnormal muscle tone (either too high or too low) are also common.

Rett syndrome is primarily caused by mutations in the MECP2 gene, located on the X chromosome. These mutations impair the function of the MECP2 protein, which plays a crucial role in brain development and function.

Since Rett syndrome is a genetic disorder, there is currently no cure. Treatment focuses on managing symptoms and providing supportive care, including physical therapy, occupational therapy, speech therapy, and specialized educational programs. Early intervention and a multidisciplinary approach involving various healthcare professionals are essential to optimize the quality of life and well-being of individuals with Rett syndrome and to provide support to their families.

Find out more about RETT SYNDROME from International Rett Syndrome Foundation

International Rett Syndrome Foundation

4500 Cooper Road, Suite 204

Blue Ash, OH 45242

(513) 874-3020

Tell Me About Smith-Magenis Syndrome

How was Smith-Magenis syndrome discovered?

Smith-Magenis syndrome (SMS) was discovered and named after the two American researchers who independently identified and characterized the disorder.

In 1982, Ann C. M. Smith, a genetic counselor, noticed similar features in several patients she was working with at a medical genetics clinic in Omaha, Nebraska. She observed shared physical characteristics, behavioral patterns, and intellectual disability among these individuals. Recognizing the possibility of a distinct syndrome, she published her findings in 1986, describing a syndrome with multiple anomalies.

Around the same time, Ellen Magenis, a clinical geneticist at the Oregon Health & Science University, was independently investigating a family with multiple affected members displaying similar physical and developmental features. In 1986, she published a report describing a new genetic syndrome based on her observations.

Following the independent discoveries by Smith and Magenis, it became clear that they had identified the same syndrome, which subsequently came to be known as Smith-Magenis syndrome.

Smith-Magenis syndrome is a complex genetic disorder primarily caused by a deletion of a portion of chromosome 17, specifically a region containing the RAI1 gene. However, in a small percentage of cases, mutations within the RAI1 gene itself can also lead to the syndrome.

Individuals with Smith-Magenis syndrome typically exhibit distinctive facial features, developmental delays, intellectual disability, sleep disturbances, behavioral issues, self-injurious behaviors, and a characteristic behavioral profile. Additional medical and physical features may include short stature, hearing loss, heart defects, skeletal abnormalities, and obesity.

Ongoing research continues to enhance our understanding of Smith-Magenis syndrome, its genetic causes, and associated symptoms. Early diagnosis, multidisciplinary management, and support services play important roles in addressing the needs of individuals with Smith-Magenis syndrome and their families.

What is Smith-Magenis Syndrome?

Smith-Magenis syndrome (SMS) is a rare genetic disorder that affects physical and cognitive development. It is caused by a deletion of genetic material in each cell from a specific region of chromosome 17. Although this region contains multiple genes, the loss of one particular gene, RAI1, is responsible for most of the features of the condition.

Signs and symptoms

People with SMS typically have a number of physical features, including:

Brachycephaly (short head)

Wide-set eyes

Prominent ears

Small jaw

High arched palate

Hypotonia (low muscle tone)

Aggressive behavior

Self-injurious behavior

Sleep disturbances

Intellectual disability

Diagnosis

SMS is a clinical diagnosis, which means that it is made based on the child's physical features and behavior. There is no single test that can definitively diagnose SMS. However, genetic testing can be used to confirm the diagnosis.

Treatment

There is no cure for SMS, but there are treatments that can help to manage the symptoms and improve the quality of life for people with the disorder. These treatments may include:

Behavioral therapy: This type of therapy can help to teach people with SMS how to manage their behavior and reduce self-injurious behavior.

Medications: Medications can be used to treat sleep disturbances, aggression, and other behavioral problems.

Occupational therapy: This type of therapy can help people with SMS develop skills for daily living, such as dressing, eating, and bathing.

Physical therapy: This type of therapy can help people with SMS improve their muscle tone and coordination.

Supportive care: This type of care can help people with SMS and their families cope with the challenges of the disorder.

Prognosis

The prognosis for people with SMS varies widely. Some people with SMS are able to live relatively independent lives, while others require lifelong care. With early diagnosis and treatment, people with SMS can live long and fulfilling lives.

Research

There is ongoing research into the causes and treatment of SMS. Some promising areas of research include:

Gene therapy: Gene therapy is a new treatment that involves replacing the missing gene responsible for SMS.

Drug development: Researchers are developing new drugs to treat the behavioral problems associated with SMS.

Education and support: Researchers are developing new educational and support programs for people with SMS and their families.

Find out more about Smith-Magenis Syndrome from prisms

PRISMS, Inc

205 Van Buren Street

Suite 120 #1027

Herndon, VA 20170

Phone: 972.231.0035

Tell Me About Williams Syndrome

How was Williams Syndrome discovered?

Williams syndrome was first identified and described by New Zealand cardiologist J.C.P. Williams in 1961. Dr. Williams observed a group of patients with a distinct pattern of cardiovascular abnormalities, particularly supravalvular aortic stenosis (narrowing of the aorta), and noted that they also exhibited a unique set of facial features and intellectual disabilities.

Further investigations and studies were conducted, and in 1964, German physician A.J. Beuren independently reported a similar group of patients with the same set of characteristics. Consequently, the syndrome came to be known as Williams-Beuren syndrome.

Over time, researchers and clinicians discovered that Williams-Beuren syndrome is a complex genetic disorder caused by a microdeletion of a portion of chromosome 7, specifically at the q11.23 region. This deletion typically includes the ELN gene (which plays a role in the elasticity of blood vessels) and may involve other nearby genes.

Williams syndrome is associated with a distinctive set of physical, developmental, and cognitive features. Individuals with Williams syndrome often display a friendly and outgoing personality, along with characteristic facial features such as a broad forehead, a flattened nasal bridge, full cheeks, a wide mouth, and dental abnormalities.

Cognitive and developmental characteristics of Williams syndrome include mild to moderate intellectual disability, specific learning difficulties, delayed language development, and a particular strength in verbal and auditory memory skills. Individuals with Williams syndrome typically exhibit a heightened interest in music, sociability, and strong social and emotional connection abilities.

Although Williams syndrome is a lifelong condition, individuals with the syndrome can lead fulfilling lives with appropriate support, early intervention, and specialized education programs tailored to their unique strengths and challenges.

Since its initial discovery, extensive research has been conducted to deepen our understanding of Williams syndrome, including its genetic underpinnings, associated medical concerns, and psychosocial aspects. This ongoing research continues to contribute to improved diagnostic methods, interventions, and support for individuals with Williams syndrome and their families.

What is Williams Syndrome?

Williams syndrome (WS) is a rare genetic disorder that affects physical and cognitive development. It is caused by a microdeletion (loss of genetic material) on chromosome 7. The deletion of about 26-28 genes is responsible for the characteristic features and symptoms of Williams syndrome.

Signs and symptoms

People with Williams syndrome typically have a number of physical features, including:

Upturned nose

Wide-set eyes

Full lips

High arched palate

Dental problems

Short stature

Joint hypermobility

Cardiovascular problems, such as supravalvular aortic stenosis (SVAS)

People with Williams syndrome also typically have a number of cognitive and behavioral features, including:

Mild to moderate intellectual disability

Hypercalcemia (high levels of calcium in the blood)

Anxiety

Attention deficit hyperactivity disorder (ADHD)

Obsessive-compulsive disorder (OCD)

Social skills

Language skills

Musical ability

Diagnosis

Williams syndrome is a clinical diagnosis, which means that it is made based on the child's physical features and behavior. There is no single test that can definitively diagnose WS. However, genetic testing can be used to confirm the diagnosis.

Treatment

There is no cure for Williams syndrome, but there are treatments that can help to manage the symptoms and improve the quality of life for people with the disorder. These treatments may include:

Cardiovascular care: People with Williams syndrome are at risk for cardiovascular problems, such as SVAS. They should be monitored by a cardiologist and may need surgery to correct the problem.

Management of hypercalcemia: People with Williams syndrome are at risk for hypercalcemia. This can be managed with medication and diet.

Behavioral therapy: Behavioral therapy can help people with Williams syndrome manage anxiety, ADHD, OCD, and other behavioral problems.

Occupational therapy: Occupational therapy can help people with Williams syndrome develop skills for daily living, such as dressing, eating, and bathing.

Physical therapy: Physical therapy can help people with Williams syndrome improve their muscle tone and coordination.

Supportive care: Supportive care can help people with Williams syndrome and their families cope with the challenges of the disorder.

Prognosis

The prognosis for people with Williams syndrome varies widely. Some people with Williams syndrome are able to live relatively independent lives, while others require lifelong care. With early diagnosis and treatment, people with Williams syndrome can live long and fulfilling lives.

Research

There is ongoing research into the causes and treatment of Williams syndrome. Some promising areas of research include:

Gene therapy: Gene therapy is a new treatment that involves replacing the missing genes responsible for Williams syndrome.

Drug development: Researchers are developing new drugs to treat the cardiovascular problems, hypercalcemia, and other medical problems associated with Williams syndrome.

Education and support: Researchers are developing new educational and support programs for people with Williams syndrome and their families.

Find out more information about Williams Syndrome from williamsyndrome Association

William Syndrome Association

243 Broadway #9188

Newark, NJ 07104

248.244.2229

800.806.1871

248.244.2230 fax

Tell Me About Cystic Fibrosis

How was Cystic Fibrosis discovered?

Cystic fibrosis (CF) was first recognized as a distinct clinical entity in the 1930s and 1940s, but the understanding of its cause and underlying mechanisms took several decades to develop.

In the early 20th century, children with CF were often diagnosed with "cystic fibrosis of the pancreas" due to the characteristic pancreatic abnormalities seen in the disease. However, the true nature of CF as a multi-organ disorder was not fully appreciated until later.

In 1936, Dr. Dorothy Andersen, an American pathologist, made significant contributions to the understanding of CF. She described the characteristic changes in the pancreas, lungs, and other organs of individuals with CF, highlighting the presence of thick mucus in the airways and pancreatic ducts.

It wasn't until the late 1980s that the underlying genetic cause of CF was discovered. In 1989, researchers at the Hospital for Sick Children in Toronto, Canada, led by Dr. Lap-Chee Tsui, identified the CFTR gene (Cystic Fibrosis Transmembrane Conductance Regulator) located on chromosome 7. Mutations in the CFTR gene were found to be responsible for the development of CF.

The CFTR gene provides instructions for producing a protein that regulates the movement of salt and water in and out of cells. Mutations in the CFTR gene result in a defective or absent CFTR protein, leading to the production of thick, sticky mucus in various organs, particularly the lungs and digestive system.

The discovery of the CFTR gene paved the way for improved understanding, diagnosis, and treatment of CF. Today, there are over 2,000 known mutations in the CFTR gene, and genetic testing can identify specific mutations to confirm a diagnosis of CF.

Ongoing research continues to advance our understanding of CF, including the development of new therapies targeting the underlying genetic defect. Treatments for CF now focus on managing the symptoms, preventing complications, and improving the quality of life for individuals with the disease. These treatments include airway clearance techniques, medication to thin mucus, enzyme replacement therapy for pancreatic insufficiency, and targeted therapies for specific CFTR mutations.

What is Cystic Fibrosis?

Cystic fibrosis (CF) is a genetic disorder that primarily affects the lungs, digestive system, and other organs. It is caused by mutations in the CFTR (Cystic Fibrosis Transmembrane Conductance Regulator) gene, which regulates the movement of salt and water in and out of cells.

The CFTR gene mutations lead to the production of a defective or insufficient CFTR protein, resulting in the production of thick, sticky mucus in various organs. The buildup of mucus primarily affects the lungs and digestive system, causing a range of symptoms and complications.

Here are some key features and characteristics of cystic fibrosis:

Respiratory Symptoms: CF primarily affects the lungs, leading to recurrent respiratory infections, chronic cough, wheezing, and difficulty breathing. The thick mucus in the airways makes individuals with CF more susceptible to lung infections, inflammation, and progressive lung damage.

Digestive Issues: CF can affect the digestive system, leading to problems with nutrient absorption, pancreatic insufficiency, and digestive enzyme deficiencies. This can result in poor weight gain, malnutrition, fatty stools, and difficulty digesting food properly.

Salt Imbalance: CFTR gene mutations also impact the movement of salt and water in sweat glands, resulting in abnormally salty sweat. This can be detected through a sweat test, which is one of the diagnostic tests for CF.

Growth and Development: CF can affect growth and development in children due to nutrient absorption issues and increased energy requirements. Delayed puberty and reduced fertility may occur in individuals with CF.

Other Organ Involvement: CF can affect various organs, including the liver, pancreas, sinuses, and reproductive system. It can lead to liver disease, sinusitis, nasal polyps, and fertility issues.

The severity and progression of CF can vary widely among individuals, depending on the specific CFTR gene mutations they carry. Advances in medical care, early diagnosis through newborn screening, and improved treatments have increased life expectancy and quality of life for individuals with CF. However, CF remains a chronic and progressive condition, and ongoing management, including daily treatments, medications, and close medical monitoring, is necessary.

It's important for individuals with CF to receive specialized care from a multidisciplinary team of healthcare professionals experienced in managing the disease. These professionals may include pulmonologists, gastroenterologists, nutritionists, respiratory therapists, and genetic counselors.

Find out more about Cystic Fibrosis from CYSTIC FIBROSIS FOUNDATION

Cystic Fibrosis Foundation (national office)

4550 Montgomery Ave.

Suite 1100 N

Bethesda, MD 20814

Local: 301-951-4422

Toll free: 800-FIGHT-CF (800-344-4823)

Tell me about Angelman syndrome

How was Angelman Syndrome discovered?

Angelman syndrome (AS) was first identified in 1965 by Dr. Harry Angelman, a British pediatrician. Dr. Angelman observed three children who were unrelated but showed similar symptoms of severe intellectual delay, stiff, jerky gait, lack of speech, seizures, motor disorders and a happy demeanor. He described these children as "puppet children" because of their jerky movements and happy appearance.

In 1982, Dr. Charles Williams and Dr. Jaime Frias of the University of Florida College of Medicine published a paper that described the genetic basis of Angelman syndrome. They found that people with Angelman syndrome have a deletion of genetic material on chromosome 15. This deletion is responsible for the characteristic features and symptoms of Angelman syndrome.

Angelman syndrome is a rare genetic disorder that affects about 1 in 15,000 people. There is no cure for Angelman syndrome, but there are treatments that can help to manage the symptoms and improve the quality of life for people with the disorder. These treatments may include:

Physical therapy: Physical therapy can help people with Angelman syndrome improve their muscle tone and coordination.

Occupational therapy: Occupational therapy can help people with Angelman syndrome develop skills for daily living, such as dressing, eating, and bathing.

Speech therapy: Speech therapy can help people with Angelman syndrome develop their communication skills.

Behavioral therapy: Behavioral therapy can help people with Angelman syndrome manage their behavior and reduce self-injurious behavior.

Supportive care: Supportive care can help people with Angelman syndrome and their families cope with the challenges of the disorder.

With early diagnosis and treatment, people with Angelman syndrome can live long and fulfilling lives.

Here are some additional facts about Angelman syndrome:

The cause of Angelman syndrome is a deletion of genetic material on chromosome 15. There is no cure for Angelman syndrome.

Treatments for Angelman syndrome are aimed at managing the symptoms and improving the quality of life.

With early diagnosis and treatment, people with Angelman syndrome can live long and fulfilling lives.

The Angelman Syndrome Foundation is a non-profit organization that is dedicated to finding a cure for Angelman syndrome and improving the lives of people affected by the disorder. The foundation funds research, provides support to families, and raises awareness of Angelman syndrome.

If you or someone you know is affected by Angelman syndrome, please contact the Angelman Syndrome Foundation for more information and support.

What is Angelman Syndrome?

Angelman syndrome is a rare genetic disorder that primarily affects the nervous system. It was first described by Dr. Harry Angelman, a British pediatrician, in 1965. The syndrome is characterized by developmental delays, intellectual disability, speech impairments, movement and balance issues, and a unique behavioral phenotype.

Here are some key features and characteristics of Angelman syndrome:

Developmental Delays: Individuals with Angelman syndrome typically experience developmental delays, including delayed motor skills such as sitting, crawling, and walking. They may also have delayed or absent speech development.

Intellectual Disability: Intellectual disability is a defining feature of Angelman syndrome, ranging from mild to severe. Individuals with the syndrome often have significant learning difficulties and may require lifelong support and specialized education.

Speech Impairments: Most individuals with Angelman syndrome have limited or no speech. They may exhibit minimal vocalizations or rely on nonverbal communication methods, such as gestures, signs, or the use of augmentative and alternative communication (AAC) devices.

Movement and Balance Issues: Individuals with Angelman syndrome often exhibit movement and balance problems, such as jerky limb movements, hand-flapping, stiff or puppet-like movements, and an unsteady gait.

Seizures: Epilepsy is common in individuals with Angelman syndrome. Seizures typically start in early childhood, and various types of seizures can occur, including generalized tonic-clonic seizures, absence seizures, and myoclonic seizures.

Behavior and Happy Demeanor: Individuals with Angelman syndrome often display a unique behavioral profile characterized by a happy and sociable demeanor. They may have frequent laughter, be easily excitable, and exhibit hyperactivity or a short attention span. Some individuals may also have behavioral challenges, such as attention deficit hyperactivity disorder (ADHD) symptoms or sleep disturbances.

Angelman syndrome is primarily caused by a lack or dysfunction of the UBE3A (ubiquitin protein ligase E3A) gene, which is located on chromosome 15. The majority of Angelman syndrome cases (about 70-75%) result from the deletion of a portion of the maternal chromosome 15. Other cases can occur due to genetic mutations in the UBE3A gene or paternal uniparental disomy (inheriting two copies of the paternal chromosome 15).

Although there is currently no cure for Angelman syndrome, supportive care and interventions can help manage the symptoms and improve the quality of life for individuals with the condition. This may include physical therapy, speech therapy, occupational therapy, behavioral interventions, and medications to address specific symptoms like seizures or sleep disturbances. Early intervention and a multidisciplinary approach are crucial in providing optimal care for individuals with Angelman syndrome.

Find out more about Angelman Syndrome from Angelman Syndrome Foundation.

Angelman Syndrome Foundation

3015 E. New York Street

Suite A2 #285

Aurora, IL 60504

800.432.6435

Tell Me About Prader-Willi Syndrome

How was Prader-Willi Syndrome discovered?

Prader-Willi syndrome (PWS) was first identified and described by two Swiss doctors, Andrea Prader and Heinrich Willi, in 1956. The doctors independently observed a group of patients who exhibited similar physical and developmental characteristics, leading them to recognize it as a distinct syndrome.

Dr. Andrea Prader, a pediatric endocrinologist, encountered a group of children with a peculiar pattern of hypotonia (low muscle tone), small hands and feet, and an insatiable appetite leading to obesity. He published his findings in 1956, describing the syndrome as "A Syndrome of Obesity, Short Stature, and Mental Retardation in Children."

Around the same time, Dr. Heinrich Willi, a Swiss psychiatrist, also noticed a similar group of patients with hyperphagia (excessive eating) leading to obesity, cognitive impairment, and distinctive physical features. He independently published his observations in 1956, describing the syndrome as "Hyperphagia-Hypogenitalism Syndrome."

Upon recognizing the overlap in their findings, Prader and Willi collaborated and jointly published a comprehensive report in 1956, establishing Prader-Willi syndrome as a distinct clinical entity. The syndrome was named after the two physicians who made significant contributions to its characterization.

Prader-Willi syndrome is a complex genetic disorder caused by the loss of genetic material in a specific region of chromosome 15. This loss of genetic material can occur in different ways, including a deletion of the paternal copy of the chromosome 15, uniparental disomy (inheritance of two copies of the chromosome from one parent), or other genetic abnormalities affecting the imprinting of genes in this region.

Individuals with Prader-Willi syndrome exhibit a range of physical, developmental, and behavioral characteristics. Some key features of Prader-Willi syndrome include early feeding difficulties in infancy, hypotonia, developmental delays, short stature, cognitive impairment, behavioral problems, and a chronic feeling of hunger that can lead to severe obesity if not managed. Individuals with PWS may also experience hormonal imbalances, sleep disturbances, and psychiatric issues.

Early diagnosis, comprehensive medical management, and a multidisciplinary approach involving healthcare professionals from various specialties are essential in providing optimal care for individuals with Prader-Willi syndrome. Treatment strategies primarily focus on managing the symptoms, including controlled diets, growth hormone therapy, behavioral interventions, and addressing associated medical conditions.

What is Prader-Willi Syndrome?

Prader-Willi syndrome (PWS) is a complex genetic disorder that affects various aspects of physical, cognitive, and behavioral development. It is caused by a genetic abnormality in chromosome 15, resulting in the loss of genetic material or disruptions in gene expression.

Here are some key characteristics and features of Prader-Willi syndrome:

Hypotonia (Low Muscle Tone): Infants with PWS often have weak muscle tone, which can lead to difficulties with sucking and feeding during early infancy.

Feeding Difficulties: In the first few years of life, individuals with PWS may experience feeding difficulties, which can be marked by poor weight gain and a failure to thrive. However, after this initial phase, they develop an insatiable appetite and a constant feeling of hunger.

Obesity and Metabolic Issues: The chronic feeling of hunger combined with a slower metabolic rate makes individuals with PWS prone to obesity. Obesity, if not managed carefully, can lead to various health problems such as diabetes, cardiovascular issues, and respiratory difficulties.

Cognitive and Intellectual Challenges: Individuals with PWS typically have mild to moderate intellectual disability. They may have learning difficulties, delayed development of speech and language skills, and exhibit impairments in executive functions and problem-solving abilities.

Behavioral and Psychiatric Characteristics: PWS is often associated with distinctive behavioral features. Individuals may have behavioral problems, including stubbornness, temper outbursts, obsessive-compulsive tendencies, and a tendency to hoard or exhibit compulsive behaviors. They may also experience mood disorders, anxiety, and a vulnerability to emotional stress.

Physical Features: Some physical characteristics commonly seen in individuals with PWS include a short stature, small hands and feet, narrow forehead, almond-shaped eyes, a thin upper lip, and a curved spine (scoliosis).

The severity and specific manifestations of Prader-Willi syndrome can vary among individuals, even within the same family. The syndrome is typically diagnosed through genetic testing, which identifies abnormalities in chromosome 15.

While there is currently no cure for Prader-Willi syndrome, management focuses on addressing the symptoms and associated medical conditions. This involves a multidisciplinary approach, including dietary management to control calorie intake, growth hormone therapy to improve growth and body composition, behavioral interventions to address compulsive behaviors and improve social skills, and monitoring and treatment of associated medical issues.

Early Intervention and ongoing support from healthcare professionals, therapists, and educators are important to help individuals with PWS reach their full potential and improve their quality of life.

Find out more about Prader-Willi Syndromed from Prader-Willi.

PWSA USA

1032 E Brandon Blvd #4744

Brandon, FL 33511

Phone: (941) 312-0400

Tell Me About Klinefelter Syndrome

How was Klinefelter Syndrome Associates discovered?

Klinefelter syndrome (KS) was first described in 1942 by Harry Klinefelter, a British physician, and his colleagues. Klinefelter observed a group of men who had small testicles, infertility, and gynecomastia (breast development). He found that these men had an extra X chromosome, resulting in a karyotype of 47,XXY.

In the years since Klinefelter's initial description, much has been learned about KS. It is now known that KS is the most common sex chromosome disorder, affecting about 1 in 500 males. KS is caused by an extra X chromosome, which can be inherited from the mother or father, or it can occur spontaneously.

KS can cause a variety of physical and hormonal symptoms, including:

Small testicles

Infertility

Gynecomastia (breast development)

Tall stature

Long limbs

High-pitched voice

Reduced muscle mass

Increased body fat

Learning disabilities

Behavioral problems

KS can also increase the risk of certain health problems, including:

Heart disease

Stroke

Diabetes

Cancer

There is no cure for KS, but there are treatments that can help to manage the symptoms and improve the quality of life. Treatment for KS may include:

Testosterone therapy: Testosterone therapy can help to restore the male sex hormones and improve the physical symptoms of KS.

Fertility treatment: There are a variety of fertility treatments that can help men with KS to father children.

Counseling: Counseling can help men with KS and their families to cope with the emotional and psychological challenges of the disorder.

With early diagnosis and treatment, men with KS can live long and fulfilling lives.

Here are some additional facts about Klinefelter syndrome:

The cause of Klinefelter syndrome is an extra X chromosome.

There is no cure for Klinefelter syndrome.

Treatments for Klinefelter syndrome are aimed at managing the symptoms and improving the quality of life.

With early diagnosis and treatment, men with Klinefelter syndrome can live long and fulfilling lives.

The Klinefelter Syndrome Association is a non-profit organization that is dedicated to providing support and information to people affected by Klinefelter syndrome. The association offers a variety of resources, including a website, support groups, and educational materials.

If you or someone you know is affected by Klinefelter syndrome, please contact the Klinefelter Syndrome Association for more information and support.

What is Klinefelter Syndrome?

Klinefelter syndrome, also known as XXY syndrome, is a genetic condition that occurs in males. It is characterized by the presence of an additional X chromosome, resulting in a chromosomal configuration of XXY instead of the typical XY.

Typically, males have one X chromosome and one Y chromosome (XY). In Klinefelter syndrome, an extra X chromosome is present, resulting in a karyotype of 47,XXY. This additional chromosome can cause a range of physical, developmental, and reproductive differences.

Here are some key features and characteristics associated with Klinefelter syndrome:

Physical Characteristics: Individuals with Klinefelter syndrome may have certain physical traits that can vary in severity. These may include tall stature, long limbs, reduced muscle tone, gynecomastia (enlarged breast tissue), broader hips, smaller testes, sparse facial and body hair, and a tendency toward obesity.

Infertility: One of the most significant effects of Klinefelter syndrome is infertility. The presence of the extra X chromosome disrupts the development of the testes, leading to reduced testosterone production and impaired sperm production. However, assisted reproductive techniques may offer options for fertility treatment.

Hormonal Imbalances: Individuals with Klinefelter syndrome may experience hormonal imbalances, including lower levels of testosterone. This can contribute to physical changes, such as reduced muscle mass, decreased bone density, and delayed or incomplete puberty.

Cognitive and Behavioral Characteristics: Some individuals with Klinefelter syndrome may have mild cognitive and learning difficulties, particularly in language and reading skills. They may also exhibit certain behavioral traits, such as shyness, social anxiety, and difficulties with social interactions.

Health Concerns: Individuals with Klinefelter syndrome may be at an increased risk for certain health conditions. These can include autoimmune disorders, metabolic issues (such as diabetes and obesity), cardiovascular problems, osteoporosis, and an increased risk of certain cancers (such as breast cancer).

Klinefelter syndrome is typically diagnosed through genetic testing, which examines the chromosomal composition. Early diagnosis is beneficial in order to provide appropriate medical care and interventions to address specific needs.

Management of Klinefelter syndrome involves a multidisciplinary approach, including regular medical monitoring, hormonal replacement therapy (testosterone), educational support, speech and language therapy if needed, and psychological support to address emotional and social challenges.

With appropriate care and support, individuals with Klinefelter syndrome can lead fulfilling lives, achieve their potential, and effectively manage associated health concerns.

Find out more about Klinefelter Syndrome from AXYS.

AXYS

PO Box 659

Paoli, PA 19301

267-338-4262

Tell me about Duchenne Muscular Dystrophy

How was Duchenne muscular dystrophy discovered?

Duchenne muscular dystrophy (DMD) was first described by the French neurologist Guillaume Benjamin Amand Duchenne in 1861. He described a group of boys who had progressive muscle weakness and wasting, and who eventually died in their teens or early twenties. Duchenne named the condition after himself.

In the early 1980s, a team of researchers led by Louis Kunkel at Boston Children's Hospital identified the gene that causes DMD. The gene is located on the X chromosome, and it is the largest gene in the human genome. Mutations in the DMD gene prevent the production of a protein called dystrophin. Dystrophin is essential for the structural integrity of muscle cells, and its absence leads to progressive muscle weakness and wasting.

Since the discovery of the DMD gene, there has been significant progress in understanding the disease and developing new treatments. There is currently no cure for DMD, but there are a number of therapies that can help to improve the quality of life for people with the condition.

Here is a timeline of the key events in the discovery of Duchenne muscular dystrophy:

1861: Guillaume Benjamin Amand Duchenne describes the condition that would later be named after him.

1986: Louis Kunkel and his team at Boston Children's Hospital identify the gene that causes DMD.

1987: The protein associated with the DMD gene is identified and named dystrophin.

1990s: The first gene therapy trials for DMD are conducted.

2000s: New drugs are developed that can help to improve muscle strength and function in people with DMD.

2010s: Gene editing technologies, such as CRISPR-Cas9, are being explored as a potential treatment for DMD.

The discovery of the DMD gene and the development of new therapies have led to significant progress in the fight against this devastating disease. However, there is still much work to be done. Researchers are working to develop more effective treatments and to find a cure for DMD.

What is Duchenne muscular dystrophy?

Duchenne muscular dystrophy (DMD) is a genetic disorder characterized by progressive muscle degeneration and weakness. It is one of the most common types of muscular dystrophy and primarily affects males, although in rare cases it can also occur in females.

DMD is caused by mutations in the gene that encodes for the protein dystrophin, which is necessary for maintaining the structural integrity of muscle fibers. Without functional dystrophin, muscle cells become fragile and are easily damaged during muscle contraction. Over time, the repeated damage and regeneration of muscle tissue lead to the replacement of muscle fibers with fibrotic (scar) tissue and fatty deposits, resulting in a gradual loss of muscle strength and function.

The symptoms of Duchenne muscular dystrophy usually become noticeable in early childhood. Children with DMD may have delayed motor skills development, difficulty walking, frequent falls, and progressive muscle weakness. As the disease progresses, they may require assistive devices like braces, wheelchairs, or scooters to aid mobility. DMD also affects the muscles involved in breathing and cardiac function, leading to respiratory and heart problems in the later stages.

Duchenne muscular dystrophy is a lifelong condition with no known cure. However, advancements in medical care, including corticosteroid medications and supportive therapies, have improved the quality of life and prolonged survival for individuals with DMD. Ongoing research and clinical trials are focused on developing novel treatments, such as gene therapy and exon-skipping therapies, that aim to address the underlying genetic cause of the disease.

Find out more about Duchenne muscular dystrophy from Parent Project Muscular Dystrophy

Parent Project Muscular Dystrophy

1012 14th Street, NW, Suite 500, Washington, DC 20005

1-800-714-5437

Tell me about Huntington's disease

Tell me about Huntington's disease

How was Huntington's disease discovered?

Huntington's disease was first described and identified by an American physician named George Huntington in 1872. Dr. Huntington observed and documented the disease in several generations of a family living in East Hampton, Long Island, New York. He referred to the condition as "chorea" due to the characteristic involuntary movements seen in affected individuals.

Dr. Huntington's initial observations and subsequent studies led to the recognition of the disease as a distinct neurological disorder. He published his findings in a medical journal titled "On Chorea" in 1872, bringing attention to the unique clinical features and hereditary nature of the condition.

Over time, more research was conducted to understand the underlying cause and genetic basis of Huntington's disease. In the late 20th century, advances in genetic technology allowed scientists to identify the specific mutation responsible for the disease. In 1993, the huntingtin gene (HTT) was discovered, and it was found that an abnormal expansion of a repeated sequence of the CAG nucleotide in this gene is the cause of Huntington's disease.

Since then, further research has been conducted to unravel the molecular mechanisms and pathology associated with the disease, leading to a better understanding of its progression and potential treatment options. Today, Huntington's disease remains an area of active scientific investigation, with ongoing efforts to develop therapies that can slow down or alleviate its symptoms.

What is Huntington's Disease?

Huntington's disease (HD) is a genetic disorder that causes progressive breakdown (degeneration) of nerve cells in the brain. Huntington's disease has a wide impact on a person's functional abilities and usually results in movement, thinking (cognitive) and psychiatric disorders.

Symptoms

The symptoms of Huntington's disease usually begin between the ages of 30 and 50, but they can appear earlier or later in life. The initial symptoms are often subtle and may include:

Mood changes, such as irritability, depression, and anxiety

Changes in personality, such as impulsiveness, poor judgment, and difficulty controlling anger

Difficulty concentrating and making decisions

Uncoordinated movements, such as involuntary twitching or jerking of the limbs

As the disease progresses, the symptoms become more severe and may include:

Severe involuntary movements, such as chorea (dance-like movements)

Difficulty walking, speaking, and swallowing

Dementia, which is a decline in thinking and memory skills

Psychiatric problems, such as psychosis (loss of contact with reality) and depression

Causes

Huntington's disease is caused by a mutation in a gene called Huntingtin. This gene is responsible for producing a protein called huntingtin. The mutation in the Huntingtin gene causes the huntingtin protein to become abnormally long. This long protein is toxic to nerve cells, and it eventually leads to their death.

Diagnosis

There is no single test that can definitively diagnose Huntington's disease. However, a doctor can often make a diagnosis based on a person's medical history, family history, and physical and neurological examinations. Genetic testing can also be used to confirm the diagnosis.

Treatment

There is no cure for Huntington's disease, but there are treatments that can help to manage the symptoms. These treatments include:

Medications to control involuntary movements, mood disorders, and psychiatric problems

Physical therapy to help improve coordination and balance

Speech therapy to help improve communication skills

Occupational therapy to help with activities of daily living

Support groups and counseling to help people cope with the emotional and psychological effects of the disease

Prognosis

The life expectancy of people with Huntington's disease is typically 15 to 20 years after the onset of symptoms. However, some people with the disease live for 30 or more years. The course of the disease varies from person to person, but it is generally progressive and worsens over time.

Research

There is ongoing research into new treatments for Huntington's disease. Some promising areas of research include gene therapy, stem cell therapy, and drug development.

Find out more about Huntington's Disease from Huntington's Disease Society of America

Huntington's Disease Society of America

505 Eighth Avenue / Suite 902

New York, NY 10018

800 345 4372

Tell me about Fragile X syndrome

How was Fragile X syndrome discovered?

Fragile X syndrome was first discovered in 1943 by Dr. Julia Bell and Dr. James Purdon Martin. They were studying a family in which a number of male members had intellectual disabilities. The men in the family also had physical features that were similar to each other, such as large heads, prominent ears, and long faces. Dr. Bell and Dr. Martin called this condition "Martin-Bell syndrome."

In 1969, Dr. Herbert Lubs made the observation of a characteristic fragile site on the lower end of the X chromosome. This fragile site was found in people with Martin-Bell syndrome. The fragile site is caused by a mutation in the Fragile X mental retardation 1 (FMR1) gene. The FMR1 gene is responsible for producing a protein called FMRP. FMRP is essential for normal brain development.

The discovery of the FMR1 gene led to a better understanding of Fragile X syndrome. It is now known that Fragile X syndrome is the most common inherited cause of intellectual disabilities in males. The syndrome can also occur in females, but it is less severe.

There is no cure for Fragile X syndrome, but there are treatments that can help to improve the symptoms. These treatments include:

Early intervention programs to help children with Fragile X syndrome reach their full potential

Medications to treat the behavioral and emotional problems that can be associated with Fragile X syndrome

Speech therapy to help improve communication skills

Occupational therapy to help with activities of daily living

Support groups and counseling to help people with Fragile X syndrome and their families cope with the challenges of the condition

Research is ongoing to find new treatments for Fragile X syndrome. Some promising areas of research include gene therapy and drug development.

What is Fragile X syndrome?

Fragile X syndrome is a genetic disorder that is one of the most common causes of inherited intellectual disability. It is also a leading cause of autism spectrum disorder (ASD) and other developmental disorders. The syndrome is characterized by a range of physical, behavioral, and cognitive symptoms.

Fragile X syndrome is caused by a mutation in the FMR1 gene located on the X chromosome. The mutation leads to the expansion of a specific sequence of DNA called CGG repeats. Normally, this sequence is repeated between 5 and 44 times. However, in individuals with Fragile X syndrome, the CGG repeats are expanded to more than 200 times, which triggers certain molecular changes in the gene.

The expanded CGG repeats in the FMR1 gene result in the reduced production or absence of a protein called fragile X mental retardation protein (FMRP). FMRP plays a crucial role in the development and functioning of the brain. Its deficiency disrupts the communication between nerve cells and affects the regulation of protein synthesis, which leads to the cognitive and behavioral impairments associated with Fragile X syndrome.

Symptoms of Fragile X syndrome can vary widely in severity and may include:

Intellectual disability: Ranging from mild to severe, intellectual disability is a common feature of Fragile X syndrome. It affects cognitive abilities, learning, and adaptive behaviors.

Behavioral and emotional challenges: Individuals with Fragile X syndrome may exhibit social anxiety, hyperactivity, attention deficits, impulsive behavior, sensory sensitivities, and emotional instability.

Physical features: Some individuals may have physical characteristics associated with the syndrome, such as a long and narrow face, large ears, a prominent forehead, and soft connective tissue.

Language and communication difficulties: Speech and language delays are common, and individuals may have trouble with articulation, expressive language, and understanding complex language.

It's important to note that not everyone with Fragile X syndrome will exhibit all of these symptoms, and the severity can vary widely among individuals. Genetic testing, typically through a blood sample, can confirm the diagnosis of Fragile X syndrome.

While there is no cure for Fragile X syndrome, management involves supportive therapies and interventions. These may include educational support, speech and language therapy, occupational therapy, behavioral interventions, and medications to address specific symptoms.

Research is ongoing to better understand Fragile X syndrome and develop potential treatments aimed at addressing the underlying molecular and cellular mechanisms associated with the disorder.

Learn more about Fragile X Syndrome from National Fragile X Foundation

Tell me about Hemophilia

How was Hemophilia discovered?

Hemophilia was not discovered in the conventional sense. Instead, its history can be traced back to ancient times when the symptoms and inheritance patterns of the disorder were observed. The condition was characterized by a tendency to bleed excessively and difficulty in clotting blood.

The earliest documented cases of hemophilia can be found in both ancient Jewish and Islamic texts. In the 2nd century AD, the Jewish Talmud described male infants dying from excessive bleeding after circumcision, which is now understood to be a manifestation of hemophilia. Similarly, in the 9th century, Islamic scholars documented cases of males from certain families experiencing severe bleeding after minor injuries or surgeries.

However, it was not until the 19th century that the modern understanding of hemophilia began to take shape. In 1803, a Philadelphia physician named John Conrad Otto published a report on a family with a bleeding disorder. He recognized that this disorder was passed down through generations and predominantly affected males. Otto referred to the condition as "bleeders' disease."

Then, in 1828, a renowned British physician named Thomas Bateman published a comprehensive description of several generations of a family affected by a bleeding disorder. He recognized the hereditary nature of the disease and coined the term "hemophilia."

Further advancements in understanding hemophilia occurred in the 20th century. In the early 20th century, scientists discovered that blood transfusions from healthy individuals could temporarily alleviate the symptoms of hemophilia. Later, in the 1950s, researchers discovered that hemophilia is caused by a deficiency or dysfunction of specific clotting factors. Hemophilia A, the most common type, was found to result from a deficiency of clotting factor VIII, while Hemophilia B resulted from a deficiency of clotting factor IX.

With the advancement of modern genetic techniques, the specific genes responsible for hemophilia were identified in the late 20th century. In 1984, the gene for factor VIII (F8) was discovered, and in 1986, the gene for factor IX (F9) was identified. This knowledge has led to improved diagnostics, genetic counseling, and the development of more targeted treatments for hemophilia.

Today, hemophilia is well understood, and ongoing research continues to advance our knowledge of the disorder, improve treatment options, and enhance the quality of life for individuals living with hemophilia.

What is Hemophilia?

Hemophilia is a rare genetic disorder that affects the blood's ability to clot. People with hemophilia have a deficiency of one or more clotting factors, which are proteins that help blood clot. This can lead to excessive bleeding after even a minor injury.

There are two main types of hemophilia: hemophilia A and hemophilia B. Hemophilia A is caused by a deficiency of factor VIII, while hemophilia B is caused by a deficiency of factor IX.

Hemophilia is inherited in an X-linked recessive manner. This means that a person must inherit two copies of the defective gene, one from each parent, in order to have the disorder. Females can be carriers of the defective gene, but they will not usually show symptoms of hemophilia unless they have two copies of the gene.

The severity of hemophilia can vary from person to person. People with severe hemophilia have very low levels of clotting factors and may bleed excessively even from minor injuries. People with moderate hemophilia have intermediate levels of clotting factors and may bleed more than normal after injuries, but they may not bleed excessively. People with mild hemophilia have higher levels of clotting factors and may only bleed excessively after major injuries or surgery.

There is no cure for hemophilia, but there are treatments that can help to prevent or control bleeding. These treatments include:

Factor replacement therapy: This is the most common treatment for hemophilia. It involves injecting the missing clotting factor into the bloodstream.

Prophylactic therapy: This is a preventive treatment that involves injecting factor VIII or IX on a regular basis to prevent bleeding.

Desmopressin (DDAVP): This is a medication that can be used to increase the body's production of clotting factors.

Platelet transfusions: This is a treatment that involves transfusing platelets into the bloodstream. Platelets are cell fragments that help to clot blood.

With proper treatment, people with hemophilia can live long and healthy lives. However, they will need to be careful to avoid activities that could lead to bleeding, such as contact sports and strenuous exercise. They will also need to be aware of the signs and symptoms of bleeding and seek medical attention promptly if they do bleed.

There is ongoing research into new treatments for hemophilia. Some promising areas of research include gene therapy and stem cell therapy.

Learn more about Hemophelia from the National Hemophilia Foundation

NHF Office Address

7 Penn Plaza Suite 1204,

New York, NY 10001, United States

Phone: 212.328.3700

Toll-free Number: 888.463.6643

Tell me about Sickle cell disease

How was Sickle cell disease discovered?

Sickle cell disease was first described and discovered in the early 20th century. The initial observations and understanding of the disease were made by multiple researchers independently.

In 1904, a Chicago physician named James Herrick made the first significant observation related to sickle cell disease. He reported on a patient of African descent who had anemia and unusual-shaped red blood cells under the microscope. The cells appeared sickle-shaped instead of the normal round shape. This marked the first recognition of the distinct abnormality in the red blood cells associated with the disease.

In subsequent years, other researchers made important contributions to the understanding of sickle cell disease. In 1910, a pathologist named E. V. Irons reported on autopsy findings of a sickle cell disease patient and noted the presence of sickle-shaped red blood cells in various tissues of the body.

Further investigations and research were conducted in the 20th century to unravel the genetic basis and underlying mechanisms of sickle cell disease. In the 1940s, it was discovered that sickle cell disease follows an autosomal recessive inheritance pattern. This means that individuals need to inherit two copies of the mutated gene, one from each parent, to develop the disease.

In 1949, Linus Pauling, an American chemist, and his colleagues identified a molecular abnormality in hemoglobin, the protein responsible for carrying oxygen in red blood cells. They found that individuals with sickle cell disease had a mutation in the gene encoding the beta-globin subunit of hemoglobin. This mutation caused a substitution of a single amino acid, resulting in the formation of abnormal hemoglobin known as hemoglobin S.

The discovery of the specific genetic mutation underlying sickle cell disease paved the way for further understanding of the disease's molecular and cellular mechanisms. It also led to the development of diagnostic tests, genetic counseling, and advances in the treatment and management of sickle cell disease.

Since then, ongoing research and medical advancements have improved our understanding of sickle cell disease, leading to better strategies for prevention, early detection, and treatment of complications associated with the condition.

What is Sickle cell disease?

Sickle cell disease (SCD) is a genetic blood disorder characterized by the presence of abnormal hemoglobin in red blood cells. It is an inherited condition that primarily affects people of African, Mediterranean, Middle Eastern, and South Asian descent.

In sickle cell disease, a mutation in the hemoglobin gene leads to the production of an abnormal form of hemoglobin called hemoglobin S (HbS). Hemoglobin is the protein in red blood cells that carries oxygen throughout the body. The presence of HbS causes red blood cells to become stiff, sticky, and misshapen, resembling a crescent or sickle shape.

The abnormal sickle-shaped red blood cells are prone to clumping together, leading to the blockage of blood flow in small blood vessels. This can cause episodes of severe pain known as "sickle cell crises" and result in damage to various organs and tissues.

Common signs and symptoms of sickle cell disease include:

Pain crises: Intense, severe pain that can occur in various body parts, such as the chest, back, abdomen, joints, and bones. These crises can last for hours to days.

Anemia: Sickle cell disease can cause chronic anemia, leading to fatigue, weakness, and shortness of breath.

Organ damage: Sickle cells can block blood vessels, leading to damage in organs such as the spleen, liver, kidneys, lungs, and brain. This can result in complications like organ failure, stroke, and pulmonary hypertension.

Infections: Individuals with sickle cell disease are more susceptible to infections, particularly those caused by bacteria that commonly affect the respiratory or urinary systems.

Delayed growth and development: Sickle cell disease can impact growth and development in children, leading to delayed puberty and stunted growth.

Eye problems: Sickle cell disease may cause damage to the blood vessels in the eyes, leading to vision problems or even blindness.

The severity of sickle cell disease varies among individuals. Some individuals may have mild symptoms, while others may experience frequent and severe complications.

Treatment for sickle cell disease aims to manage symptoms, prevent complications, and improve quality of life. This may include medications to relieve pain, manage infections, and prevent complications like strokes. Blood transfusions, supplemental oxygen, and bone marrow transplants may also be utilized in certain cases.

Recent advancements in treatments, such as gene therapies and targeted medications, offer promising prospects for the future management of sickle cell disease. Regular medical check-ups, proactive management of symptoms, and a healthy lifestyle are important for individuals with sickle cell disease to minimize complications and maintain overall well-being.

Learn more about Sickle Cell Disease from Sickle Cell Disease Association of America

Sickle Cell Disease Association of America

7240 Parkway Drive, Suite 180

Hanover, Maryland 21076

410.528.1555 (office)

410.528.1495 (fax)

800.421.8453 (toll-free)

Tell me about Tay-Sachs disease

How was Tay-Sachs disease discovered?

1

Tay-Sachs disease was discovered in 1881 by British ophthalmologist Warren Tay and American neurologist Bernard Sachs. Tay described a cherry-red spot on the retina of the eye in a one-year-old patient, and Sachs described the cellular changes of Tay-Sachs and noted an increased prevalence in the Eastern European Jewish (Ashkenazi) population in 1887.

Tay-Sachs disease is a rare, inherited disorder that causes progressive damage to the nervous system. It is caused by a mutation in the HEXA gene, which is responsible for producing an enzyme called hexosaminidase A. Hexosaminidase A breaks down a fatty substance called GM2 ganglioside, which is normally found in the brain. In people with Tay-Sachs disease, hexosaminidase A is not produced or is not produced in sufficient amounts. This leads to the buildup of GM2 ganglioside in the brain, which damages nerve cells and eventually leads to death.

Tay-Sachs disease is a fatal disorder. Most children with Tay-Sachs disease die by the age of 4. There is no cure for Tay-Sachs disease, but there are treatments that can help to manage the symptoms. These treatments include:

Steroid therapy: Steroids can help to reduce inflammation in the brain and improve symptoms.

Bone marrow transplantation: Bone marrow transplantation is a procedure in which healthy bone marrow cells are transplanted into the body of a person with Tay-Sachs disease. This procedure can help to improve the symptoms of Tay-Sachs disease, but it is not a cure.

What is Tay-Sachs disease?

Tay-Sachs disease is a rare genetic disorder characterized by the progressive destruction of nerve cells in the brain and spinal cord. It is named after two physicians, Warren Tay and Bernard Sachs, who independently described the disease in the late 19th and early 20th centuries, respectively.

Tay-Sachs disease is caused by a genetic mutation that affects the production of an enzyme called hexosaminidase-A (Hex-A). This enzyme plays a vital role in breaking down a fatty substance called GM2 ganglioside, which accumulates in nerve cells in individuals with Tay-Sachs disease.

The disease is inherited in an autosomal recessive manner, meaning that an individual must inherit two copies of the mutated gene (one from each parent) to develop the disorder. The mutated gene responsible for Tay-Sachs disease is called HEXA and is located on chromosome 15.

Tay-Sachs disease primarily affects the nervous system, and symptoms typically appear in infancy or early childhood. The early-onset form, known as infantile Tay-Sachs disease, is the most common and severe type. Infants with the disease initially appear normal but start showing signs of developmental regression around 3 to 6 months of age. Symptoms may include:

Loss of motor skills: Infants gradually lose their ability to crawl, sit, and eventually become immobile.

Excessive startle response: The Moro reflex, an exaggerated startle reflex, becomes prominent.

Weakness and muscle stiffness: Muscle tone decreases, leading to muscle weakness and stiffness (hypertonia).

Vision and hearing problems: Loss of vision and hearing abilities may occur.

Seizures: Infants may experience seizures, which can be frequent and severe.

Swallowing difficulties: Difficulties with feeding and swallowing can arise.

The progression of the disease is relentless, and affected infants typically experience severe neurological decline. Sadly, the prognosis is generally poor, and most children with infantile Tay-Sachs disease do not survive beyond early childhood.

Less commonly, there are rarer forms of Tay-Sachs disease with later onset, including juvenile and adult forms. These forms tend to have slower disease progression and milder symptoms, but still result in neurological deterioration over time.

Currently, there is no cure for Tay-Sachs disease. Treatment focuses on managing symptoms and providing supportive care. Genetic counseling and prenatal testing are available for families at risk of having a child with Tay-Sachs disease to help with family planning and early detection. Research continues to advance our understanding of the disease and explore potential therapeutic approaches.

Learn more about Tay-Sachs Disease from National Tay-Sachs & Allied Diseases Association

National Tay-Sachs & Allied Diseases Association

2001 Beacon Street, Suite 204

Boston, MA 02135

(617) 277-4463

Tell me about Niemann-Pick disease

How was Niemann-Pick disease discovered?

Niemann-Pick disease (NPD) was first described in 1914 by Albert Niemann, a German pediatrician. He described a young child with hepatosplenomegaly, a condition in which the liver and spleen are enlarged. The child also had neurological problems, including seizures and developmental delays. Niemann named the condition after himself.

In 1927, Ludwig Pick, a German pathologist, studied tissues from children who had died from Niemann-Pick disease. He found that the cells in the liver, spleen, and brain were filled with a fatty substance called sphingomyelin. Pick also found that the cells were unable to break down sphingomyelin, which led to its accumulation in the cells.

Niemann-Pick disease is a rare, inherited disorder that is caused by a mutation in the SMPD1 gene. The SMPD1 gene is responsible for producing an enzyme called acid sphingomyelinase. Acid sphingomyelinase breaks down sphingomyelin, which is a type of fat that is found in all cells in the body.

In people with Niemann-Pick disease, acid sphingomyelinase is not produced or is not produced in sufficient amounts. This leads to the accumulation of sphingomyelin in the cells, which damages the cells and eventually leads to death.

There are three types of Niemann-Pick disease: type A, type B, and type C. Type A is the most severe form of the disease. It usually begins in infancy and is fatal by the age of 4. Type B is a less severe form of the disease. It usually begins in childhood and people with type B can live into adulthood. Type C is a milder form of the disease. It usually begins in adulthood and people with type C can live normal lives.

There is no cure for Niemann-Pick disease. Treatment is aimed at managing the symptoms. Treatment options include:

Bone marrow transplantation: Bone marrow transplantation is a procedure in which healthy bone marrow cells are transplanted into the body of a person with Niemann-Pick disease. This procedure has been shown to be effective in some cases of type A Niemann-Pick disease.

Splenectomy: Splenectomy is a surgical procedure in which the spleen is removed. The spleen is a large organ that is located in the upper left abdomen. The spleen is responsible for removing old red blood cells from the bloodstream. In people with Niemann-Pick disease, the spleen can become enlarged and can cause pain and other problems. Splenectomy can help to relieve these problems.

Other treatments: Other treatments that may be used to manage the symptoms of Niemann-Pick disease include:

Medications to control seizures

Medications to improve lung function

Physical therapy

Occupational therapy

Speech therapy

Support groups

Niemann-Pick disease is a serious and life-threatening disorder. However, with early diagnosis and treatment, people with Niemann-Pick disease can live long and productive lives.

What Is Niemann-Pick disease?

Niemann-Pick disease is a group of rare genetic disorders characterized by the abnormal accumulation of lipids, particularly sphingomyelin, in various tissues and organs of the body. It is named after two physicians, Albert Niemann and Ludwig Pick, who independently described different forms of the disease.

There are several types of Niemann-Pick disease, but the most common ones are Niemann-Pick type A and Niemann-Pick type B:

Niemann-Pick type A (NPA): This is the most severe form of the disease. It is caused by a deficiency of an enzyme called acid sphingomyelinase (ASM), which leads to the buildup of sphingomyelin in cells. NPA typically presents in infancy and is characterized by progressive neurological deterioration, hepatosplenomegaly (enlarged liver and spleen), feeding difficulties, and a shortened lifespan.

Niemann-Pick type B (NPB): NPB is less severe than NPA. It is also caused by a deficiency of ASM but with residual enzyme activity. NPB primarily affects the liver, spleen, and lungs. Symptoms may include hepatosplenomegaly, respiratory problems, delayed growth, and in some cases, mild neurological involvement. NPB typically presents later in childhood or even adulthood.

Other less common forms of Niemann-Pick disease include Niemann-Pick type C (NPC). NPC is caused by mutations in either the NPC1 or NPC2 gene, leading to impaired lipid metabolism and the accumulation of lipids in various organs, including the brain. NPC is characterized by a wide range of symptoms, including neurological problems, hepatosplenomegaly, lung involvement, impaired coordination, cognitive decline, and seizures. The age of onset and disease severity can vary widely, with some cases presenting in infancy and others in adulthood.

Niemann-Pick disease is inherited in an autosomal recessive manner, meaning that an individual must inherit two copies of the mutated gene (one from each parent) to develop the disorder. Genetic testing and counseling can help identify carriers and individuals at risk of having a child with Niemann-Pick disease.

While there is currently no cure for Niemann-Pick disease, management focuses on symptomatic treatment and supportive care. This may include addressing respiratory issues, nutritional support, physical and occupational therapy, and medications to manage specific symptoms. Research is ongoing to develop potential therapies aimed at addressing the underlying genetic and metabolic abnormalities associated with the different forms of Niemann-Pick disease.

Learn more about Niemann-Pick Disease from nndpf

National Niemann Pick Disease Foundation

National Niemann-Pick disease Foundation (NNPDF)

P.O. Box 49

Fort Atkinson, WI 53538-0049

Phone: 877-287-3672

Tell me about Gaucher disease

How was Gaucher disease discovered?

Gaucher disease was first discovered in 1882 by Philippe Gaucher, a French doctor. He described a young woman with an enlarged spleen and liver. Gaucher also found that the woman's blood contained abnormal cells called Gaucher cells.

Gaucher disease is a rare, inherited disorder that is caused by a mutation in the GBA gene. The GBA gene is responsible for producing an enzyme called glucocerebrosidase. Glucocerebrosidase breaks down a fatty substance called glucocerebroside, which is normally found in all cells in the body.

In people with Gaucher disease, glucocerebrosidase is not produced or is not produced in sufficient amounts. This leads to the accumulation of glucocerebroside in the cells, which damages the cells and eventually leads to death.

There are three types of Gaucher disease: type 1, type 2, and type 3. Type 1 is the most common form of the disease. It is a chronic disorder that can cause a variety of symptoms, including anemia, bone pain, and enlarged spleen and liver. Type 2 is a much rarer form of the disease. It is a more severe form of the disease that usually leads to death in early childhood. Type 3 is a very rare form of the disease. It is a progressive disorder that usually leads to death in adolescence.

There is no cure for Gaucher disease. Treatment is aimed at managing the symptoms. Treatment options include:

Enzyme replacement therapy: Enzyme replacement therapy is a treatment in which a person with Gaucher disease is given injections of glucocerebrosidase. This treatment can help to reduce the amount of glucocerebroside in the cells and improve the symptoms of the disease.

Bone marrow transplantation: Bone marrow transplantation is a procedure in which healthy bone marrow cells are transplanted into the body of a person with Gaucher disease. This procedure has been shown to be effective in some cases of type 1 Gaucher disease.

Other treatments: Other treatments that may be used to manage the symptoms of Gaucher disease include:

Medications to control anemia

Medications to relieve bone pain

Splenectomy: Splenectomy is a surgical procedure in which the spleen is removed. The spleen is a large organ that is located in the upper left abdomen. The spleen is responsible for removing old red blood cells from the bloodstream. In people with Gaucher disease, the spleen can become enlarged and can cause pain and other problems. Splenectomy can help to relieve these problems.

Physical therapy

Occupational therapy

Speech therapy

Support groups

Gaucher disease is a serious and life-threatening disorder. However, with early diagnosis and treatment, people with Gaucher disease can live long and productive lives.

What is Gaucher disease?

Gaucher disease is a rare genetic disorder characterized by the accumulation of a fatty substance called glucocerebroside within certain cells and organs of the body, particularly the spleen, liver, and bone marrow. It is named after Philippe Gaucher, the French physician who first described the disease in 1882.

Gaucher disease is caused by mutations in the GBA gene, which provides instructions for producing an enzyme called glucocerebrosidase (also known as acid beta-glucosidase). This enzyme plays a crucial role in breaking down glucocerebroside into smaller molecules that can be processed and eliminated from the body. In Gaucher disease, the deficiency or impaired function of glucocerebrosidase leads to the accumulation of glucocerebroside in various tissues.

There are three main types of Gaucher disease:

Type 1 Gaucher disease: This is the most common form of the disease and typically affects adults. It can manifest at any age and has a wide range of symptoms and disease progression. Common symptoms may include an enlarged spleen and liver, low platelet count (thrombocytopenia), anemia, bone pain, fatigue, and an increased risk of fractures. In some cases, mild neurological involvement may occur.

Type 2 Gaucher disease: Also known as acute infantile Gaucher disease, this is a severe and rapidly progressive form of the disease that typically affects infants. Symptoms may include extensive neurological involvement, including developmental delay, seizures, muscle rigidity, breathing difficulties, and organ enlargement. Unfortunately, infants with type 2 Gaucher disease often have a significantly shortened lifespan.

Type 3 Gaucher disease: This form falls between types 1 and 2 in terms of severity and progression. Type 3 Gaucher disease can present in childhood or adulthood and features a slower disease progression than type 2. Neurological symptoms, such as ataxia (loss of muscle coordination), may occur along with the typical visceral manifestations of the disease.

Gaucher disease is inherited in an autosomal recessive manner, meaning that an individual must inherit two copies of the mutated GBA gene (one from each parent) to develop the disorder. Genetic testing and counseling can help identify carriers and individuals at risk of having a child with Gaucher disease.

Although there is no cure for Gaucher disease, there are effective treatments available. Enzyme replacement therapy (ERT) is a common treatment approach that involves intravenous infusion of a synthetic version of the missing enzyme to help break down glucocerebroside. Substrate reduction therapy (SRT) and other emerging therapeutic approaches are also being explored. These treatments aim to alleviate symptoms, reduce organ enlargement, improve blood counts, and enhance overall quality of life for individuals with Gaucher disease.

Learn more about Gaucher Disease from National Goucher Foundation

National Gaucher Foundation

5410 Edson Lane #220

Rockville, MD 20852

800-504-3189

Tell me about Pompe disease

How was Pompe disease discovered?

Pompe disease, also known as glycogen storage disease type II, is a rare genetic disorder caused by a deficiency of the enzyme acid alpha-glucosidase (GAA). The discovery and understanding of Pompe disease involved a series of scientific observations and advancements. Here is an overview of the historical developments in the discovery of Pompe disease:

Early Observations: In the early 1930s, Dr. J.C. Pompe, a Dutch pathologist, described the case of an infant who had an enlarged heart, muscle weakness, and a buildup of glycogen (a form of stored sugar) in various tissues. Dr. Pompe identified this condition as a distinct disease, which later came to be known as Pompe disease.

Recognition as a Glycogen Storage Disorder: In the subsequent years, researchers recognized Pompe disease as a type of glycogen storage disorder characterized by the abnormal accumulation of glycogen within the cells, particularly in muscle tissues. This led to the understanding that the underlying cause of Pompe disease was a deficiency of the enzyme responsible for breaking down glycogen.

Enzyme Deficiency: In the 1960s and 1970s, researchers further characterized the specific enzyme deficiency in Pompe disease. They identified the enzyme acid alpha-glucosidase (GAA) as the enzyme that is deficient or defective in individuals with Pompe disease. This deficiency leads to the accumulation of glycogen in various tissues, primarily affecting the muscles.

Genetic Basis: In the late 1990s and early 2000s, researchers discovered the genetic basis of Pompe disease. They identified mutations in the GAA gene that result in a deficiency or malfunctioning of the GAA enzyme. This understanding of the genetic cause allowed for more accurate diagnosis and genetic testing for Pompe disease.

Diagnostic and Treatment Advances: Over time, advancements in diagnostic techniques, such as enzyme assays and genetic testing, have improved the accuracy and speed of diagnosing Pompe disease. Treatment options have also advanced significantly. Enzyme replacement therapy (ERT) has become the standard treatment for Pompe disease. ERT involves intravenous infusion of the missing or deficient enzyme to help break down glycogen and prevent its buildup in tissues.

Continued Research: Ongoing research in Pompe disease focuses on understanding the disease mechanisms, developing more effective therapies, and improving patient outcomes. Scientists are exploring gene therapy approaches, next-generation enzyme replacement therapies, and other treatment modalities to further enhance the management of Pompe disease.

The discovery and ongoing research in Pompe disease have led to improved diagnostic techniques, the development of specific treatments such as enzyme replacement therapy, and ongoing advancements in understanding the underlying biology of the disease. These efforts have contributed to improved outcomes and quality of life for individuals affected by Pompe disease.

What is Pompe disease?

Pompe disease, also known as acid maltase disease or glycogen storage disease type II, is a rare genetic disorder that causes progressive weakness to the heart and skeletal muscles.

Pompe disease is caused by mutations in the GAA gene, which makes an enzyme called acid alpha-glucosidase (GAA). The GAA enzyme is responsible for breaking down glycogen, a stored form of sugar used for energy. In Pompe disease, the GAA enzyme is either missing or defective, which causes glycogen to build up in the body's cells, particularly in the heart and skeletal muscles. This buildup of glycogen can damage the cells and lead to muscle weakness and other problems.

Pompe disease is inherited in an autosomal recessive manner, which means that both parents must carry a copy of the mutated gene in order for their child to be born with the disease.

There are three types of Pompe disease:

Classic Infantile-onset Pompe disease: This is the most severe form of the disease and usually begins in the first few months of life. Infants with classic infantile-onset Pompe disease may have difficulty feeding, breathing, and moving. They may also have heart problems and seizures. Without treatment, most infants with classic infantile-onset Pompe disease die by the age of two.

Non-classic infantile-onset Pompe disease: This form of the disease is less severe than classic infantile-onset Pompe disease. Symptoms may not appear until later in childhood or even adulthood. People with non-classic infantile-onset Pompe disease may have muscle weakness, heart problems, and breathing problems. However, they often do not have seizures and they may be able to live a normal life with treatment.

Late-onset Pompe disease: This form of the disease is the least severe and usually does not appear until adulthood. People with late-onset Pompe disease may have muscle weakness, heart problems, and breathing problems. However, they often do not have seizures and they may be able to live a normal life with treatment.

There is no cure for Pompe disease, but there are treatments that can help to manage the symptoms and improve quality of life. Treatment options include:

Enzyme replacement therapy (ERT): ERT is a treatment that replaces the missing or defective GAA enzyme. ERT is given as an infusion into the bloodstream and can help to improve muscle strength and reduce the risk of heart problems.

Gene therapy: Gene therapy is a new treatment that is still in clinical trials. Gene therapy involves replacing the mutated GAA gene with a healthy copy of the gene. Gene therapy has the potential to cure Pompe disease, but it is still too early to say for sure if it will be successful.

With treatment, people with Pompe disease can live long and productive lives. However, the disease can be progressive and some people may eventually experience complications such as heart failure, respiratory failure, and kidney failure.

Learn more about Pompe disease from the United Pompe Foundation

United Pompe Foundation

David W. Hamlin

5100 N. Sixth Street #119

Fresno, CA 93710

Phone: (559) 227-1898

Tell me about Krabbe disease

How was Krabbe disease discovered?

Krabbe disease, also known as globoid cell leukodystrophy, is a rare genetic disorder that primarily affects the nervous system. The discovery and understanding of Krabbe disease involved a series of scientific observations and advancements. Here is an overview of the historical developments in the discovery of Krabbe disease:

Early Observations: Krabbe disease was first described by Dr. Knud Krabbe, a Danish neurologist, in 1916. Dr. Krabbe reported the case of an infant with neurological symptoms, including muscle weakness, developmental regression, and vision loss. The post-mortem examination revealed abnormalities in the nervous system, specifically the presence of abnormal cells called globoid cells.

Recognition as a Distinct Disorder: In the subsequent years, Krabbe disease was recognized as a distinct disorder with characteristic clinical and pathological features. It was classified as a leukodystrophy, a group of genetic disorders characterized by abnormal development or destruction of the white matter in the brain.

Genetic Basis: In the late 1960s and early 1970s, researchers made significant advancements in understanding the genetic basis of Krabbe disease. They identified a deficiency of the enzyme galactosylceramidase (GALC) as the underlying cause of the disease. This deficiency results in the accumulation of a fatty substance called psychosine, which damages the myelin sheath, the protective covering of nerve fibers.

Diagnostic Advances: Over time, diagnostic techniques for Krabbe disease have improved. The measurement of GALC enzyme activity and the analysis of genetic mutations in the GALC gene have become the standard diagnostic methods for Krabbe disease. Newborn screening programs have been implemented in some regions to identify affected infants early, allowing for early intervention and treatment.

Treatment Approaches: Although there is currently no cure for Krabbe disease, treatment options have evolved. Hematopoietic stem cell transplantation (HSCT) has shown promise in slowing the progression of the disease in some individuals, particularly if performed early in the course of the disease. HSCT aims to replace the defective cells with healthy cells that can produce the missing enzyme.

Continued Research: Ongoing research in Krabbe disease focuses on understanding the disease mechanisms, identifying potential therapeutic targets, and developing new treatment approaches. Scientists are exploring gene therapy techniques, enzyme replacement therapies, and other strategies to improve outcomes for individuals with Krabbe disease.

The discovery and ongoing research in Krabbe disease have led to improved diagnostic techniques, the implementation of newborn screening programs, and the exploration of potential treatment options. While challenges remain, these efforts contribute to advancing our understanding of the disease and improving the management and outcomes for individuals affected by Krabbe disease.

What is Krabbe disease?

Krabbe disease, also known as globoid cell leukodystrophy, is a rare, inherited disorder that affects the nervous system. It is caused by a deficiency in the enzyme galactocerebrosidase, which is responsible for breaking down a fatty substance called galactocerebroside. When this enzyme is missing or defective, galactocerebroside builds up in the brain and spinal cord, causing damage to nerve cells and leading to neurological symptoms.

Krabbe disease is a progressive disorder, meaning that it gets worse over time. Symptoms usually begin in early infancy and can include:

Seizures

Feeding problems

Vision problems

Hearing problems

Developmental delays

Stiffness

Weakness

Enlarged liver and spleen

Involuntary movements

As the disease progresses, people with Krabbe disease may experience more severe neurological problems, such as:

Paralysis

Deafness

Blindness

Mental retardation

Seizures

Death

There is no cure for Krabbe disease, but there are treatments that can help to manage the symptoms and improve quality of life. Treatment options include:

Enzyme replacement therapy (ERT): ERT is a treatment that replaces the missing or defective galactocerebrosidase enzyme. ERT is given as an infusion into the bloodstream and can help to slow the progression of the disease.

Bone marrow transplant (BMT): BMT is a procedure in which healthy stem cells are transplanted into the body of a person with Krabbe disease. BMT can help to improve neurological function and prolong life.

Supportive care: Supportive care includes measures such as feeding tube placement, respiratory support, and pain management.

The outlook for people with Krabbe disease is poor. Most people with the disease die before the age of 5. However, some people with Krabbe disease have lived into their teens or twenties with the help of treatment.

Krabbe disease is a devastating disease, but there are treatments that can help to improve quality of life. If you or your child has been diagnosed with Krabbe disease, it is important to talk to your doctor about treatment options and how to best manage the disease.

Learn more about Krabbe disease from Hunter's Hope Foundation

Hunter's Hope

PO Box 643

Orchard Park, NY 14127

(716) 667-1200

Tell me about Hunter syndrome

How was Hunter syndrome discovered?

Hunter syndrome, also known as mucopolysaccharidosis type II (MPS II), is a rare genetic disorder that primarily affects the lysosomal storage of complex carbohydrates. The discovery and understanding of Hunter syndrome involved a series of scientific observations and advancements. Here is an overview of the historical developments in the discovery of Hunter syndrome:

Clinical Observations: In the late 19th century, Dr. Charles Hunter, a Canadian physician, observed a set of symptoms in male patients that included progressive developmental delay, coarse facial features, enlarged liver and spleen, joint stiffness, and other skeletal abnormalities. Dr. Hunter documented these cases, recognizing that they represented a distinct clinical entity.

Recognition as a Distinct Disorder: In the early 20th century, additional cases with similar features were reported by other physicians, further establishing Hunter syndrome as a distinct disorder. It was classified as a mucopolysaccharidosis, a group of lysosomal storage disorders characterized by the accumulation of complex carbohydrates called mucopolysaccharides.

Biochemical Basis: In the 1960s and 1970s, researchers made significant advancements in understanding the biochemical basis of Hunter syndrome. They discovered that individuals with Hunter syndrome have a deficiency or absence of the enzyme iduronate 2-sulfatase (IDS). This enzyme is responsible for breaking down specific mucopolysaccharides called dermatan sulfate and heparan sulfate. The deficiency of IDS leads to the accumulation of these substances in various tissues, causing the characteristic symptoms of Hunter syndrome.

Genetic Discoveries: In the 1980s and 1990s, the genes associated with Hunter syndrome were identified. Researchers found that the IDS gene, located on the X chromosome, is mutated in individuals with Hunter syndrome. As an X-linked recessive disorder, Hunter syndrome primarily affects males, while females are usually carriers of the gene mutation.

Diagnostic Advances: Over time, diagnostic techniques for Hunter syndrome have improved. Measurement of IDS enzyme activity and genetic testing for mutations in the IDS gene have become standard diagnostic methods. These tests help confirm the diagnosis and determine the specific mutation involved, facilitating genetic counseling and carrier detection.

Treatment Approaches: While there is no cure for Hunter syndrome, various treatment approaches have been developed to manage the symptoms and slow disease progression. Enzyme replacement therapy (ERT) has shown promise in improving certain aspects of the disease. It involves regular infusions of a synthetic form of the missing IDS enzyme to help break down the accumulated mucopolysaccharides. Supportive care, including physical therapy, speech therapy, and medications, is also provided to manage specific symptoms.

Continued Research: Ongoing research in Hunter syndrome focuses on understanding the disease mechanisms, further improving treatment options, and exploring potential gene therapies. Scientists are investigating novel approaches, such as gene editing and stem cell-based therapies, to address the underlying genetic defect and provide more effective treatments for Hunter syndrome.

The discovery and ongoing research in Hunter syndrome have led to improved diagnostic techniques, the development of specific treatment approaches, and advancements in understanding the underlying biology of the disease. These efforts contribute to improved outcomes and quality of life for individuals affected by Hunter syndrome.

What is Hunter syndrome?

Hunter syndrome, also known as mucopolysaccharidosis type II (MPS II), is a rare genetic disorder that affects the body's ability to break down certain complex sugars. This leads to the buildup of these sugars in the body's tissues, which can cause a variety of problems, including physical and mental development delays, heart problems, and breathing problems.

Hunter syndrome is caused by a mutation in the IDS gene, which is responsible for producing an enzyme called iduronate-2-sulfatase. This enzyme is needed to break down a type of complex sugar called heparan sulfate. When the IDS gene is mutated, the body cannot produce enough iduronate-2-sulfatase, which leads to the buildup of heparan sulfate in the body.

Hunter syndrome is inherited in an X-linked recessive manner, which means that a boy must inherit the mutated gene from his mother in order to be born with the disease. Girls who inherit the mutated gene are carriers, but they do not typically show any symptoms of the disease.

The symptoms of Hunter syndrome can vary from person to person, but they typically begin in early childhood. Common symptoms include:

Physical development delays: Children with Hunter syndrome may have delayed growth and development. They may also have coarse facial features, such as a large head, prominent forehead, and thick lips.

Mental development delays: Children with Hunter syndrome may have intellectual disabilities. They may also have difficulty with speech and language.

Heart problems: Children with Hunter syndrome may have heart problems, such as enlarged heart and heart valve problems.

Breathing problems: Children with Hunter syndrome may have breathing problems, such as obstructive sleep apnea and chronic lung disease.

Other problems: Children with Hunter syndrome may also experience other problems, such as hearing loss, vision problems, and joint pain.

There is no cure for Hunter syndrome, but there are treatments that can help to manage the symptoms and improve quality of life. Treatment options include:

Enzyme replacement therapy (ERT): ERT is a treatment that replaces the missing or defective iduronate-2-sulfatase enzyme. ERT is given as an infusion into the bloodstream and can help to reduce the buildup of heparan sulfate in the body.

Gene therapy: Gene therapy is a new treatment that is still in clinical trials. Gene therapy involves replacing the mutated IDS gene with a healthy copy of the gene. Gene therapy has the potential to cure Hunter syndrome, but it is still too early to say for sure if it will be successful.

Supportive care: Supportive care includes measures such as feeding tube placement, respiratory support, and pain management.

The outlook for people with Hunter syndrome varies depending on the severity of the disease. Some people with Hunter syndrome live into their 20s or 30s, while others die in childhood. However, with treatment, people with Hunter syndrome can live long and productive lives.

If you or your child has been diagnosed with Hunter syndrome, it is important to talk to your doctor about treatment options and how to best manage the disease. There are many resources available to help people with Hunter syndrome and their families, including the Hunter Syndrome Foundation and the MPS Society.

Learn more about Hunter syndrome from the MPS Society

MPS Society, MPS House,

Repton Place, White Lion Road,

Amersham, Buckinghamshire,

HP7 9LP, United Kingdom

0345 389 9901

Tell me about Hurler syndrome

How was Hurler syndrome discovered?

Hurler syndrome, also known as mucopolysaccharidosis type I (MPS I), is a rare genetic disorder that primarily affects the lysosomal storage of complex carbohydrates. The discovery and understanding of Hurler syndrome involved a series of scientific observations and advancements. Here is an overview of the historical developments in the discovery of Hurler syndrome:

Clinical Observations: In 1919, a German physician named Gertrud Hurler first described a set of symptoms in children that included skeletal abnormalities, developmental delay, coarse facial features, and organomegaly (enlarged organs). Dr. Hurler observed a pattern among these cases, recognizing that they represented a distinct clinical entity.

Recognition as a Distinct Disorder: In subsequent years, additional cases with similar features were reported by other physicians, further establishing Hurler syndrome as a distinct disorder. It was classified as a mucopolysaccharidosis, a group of lysosomal storage disorders characterized by the accumulation of complex carbohydrates called mucopolysaccharides.

Biochemical Basis: In the 1960s and 1970s, researchers made significant advancements in understanding the biochemical basis of Hurler syndrome. They discovered that individuals with Hurler syndrome have a deficiency or absence of the enzyme alpha-L-iduronidase. This enzyme is responsible for breaking down specific mucopolysaccharides called dermatan sulfate and heparan sulfate. The deficiency of alpha-L-iduronidase leads to the accumulation of these substances in various tissues, causing the characteristic symptoms of Hurler syndrome.

Genetic Discoveries: In the 1990s, the gene associated with Hurler syndrome was identified. Researchers found that mutations in the IDUA gene, located on chromosome 4, result in a deficiency of alpha-L-iduronidase. These gene mutations are responsible for the impaired enzyme activity and subsequent mucopolysaccharide accumulation in Hurler syndrome.

Diagnostic Advances: Over time, diagnostic techniques for Hurler syndrome have improved. Measurement of alpha-L-iduronidase enzyme activity and genetic testing for mutations in the IDUA gene have become standard diagnostic methods. These tests help confirm the diagnosis and determine the specific mutation involved, facilitating genetic counseling and carrier detection.

Treatment Approaches: Although there is no cure for Hurler syndrome, various treatment approaches have been developed to manage the symptoms and slow disease progression. Hematopoietic stem cell transplantation (HSCT) has shown promise in improving certain aspects of the disease. HSCT involves replacing the patient's bone marrow with healthy donor cells that can produce the missing enzyme. Enzyme replacement therapy (ERT) is another treatment option that involves regular infusions of a synthetic form of alpha-L-iduronidase to help break down the accumulated mucopolysaccharides. Supportive care, including physical therapy, speech therapy, and surgeries, is also provided to manage specific symptoms.

Continued Research: Ongoing research in Hurler syndrome focuses on understanding the disease mechanisms, further improving treatment options, and exploring potential gene therapies. Scientists are investigating novel approaches, such as gene editing and advanced delivery methods for enzyme replacement therapy, to address the underlying genetic defect and provide more effective treatments for Hurler syndrome.

The discovery and ongoing research in Hurler syndrome have led to improved diagnostic techniques, the development of specific treatment approaches, and advancements in understanding the underlying biology of the disease. These efforts contribute to improved outcomes and quality of life for individuals affected by Hurler syndrome.

What is Hurler syndrome?

Hurler syndrome, also known as mucopolysaccharidosis type I (MPS I), is a rare genetic disorder that affects the body's ability to break down certain complex sugars. This leads to the buildup of these sugars in the body's tissues, which can cause a variety of problems, including physical and mental development delays, heart problems, and breathing problems.

Hurler syndrome is caused by a mutation in the IDUA gene, which is responsible for producing an enzyme called alpha-L-iduronidase. This enzyme is needed to break down a type of complex sugar called dermatan sulfate. When the IDUA gene is mutated, the body cannot produce enough alpha-L-iduronidase, which leads to the buildup of dermatan sulfate in the body.

Hurler syndrome is inherited in an autosomal recessive manner, which means that both parents must carry a mutated gene in order for their child to be born with the disease.

The symptoms of Hurler syndrome can vary from person to person, but they typically begin in early childhood. Common symptoms include:

Physical development delays: Children with Hurler syndrome may have delayed growth and development. They may also have coarse facial features, such as a large head, prominent forehead, and thick lips.

Mental development delays: Children with Hurler syndrome may have intellectual disabilities. They may also have difficulty with speech and language.

Heart problems: Children with Hurler syndrome may have heart problems, such as enlarged heart and heart valve problems.

Breathing problems: Children with Hurler syndrome may have breathing problems, such as obstructive sleep apnea and chronic lung disease.

Joint problems: Children with Hurler syndrome may have joint problems, such as stiffness and pain.

Hearing loss: Children with Hurler syndrome may have hearing loss.

Vision problems: Children with Hurler syndrome may have vision problems, such as clouding of the cornea.

There is no cure for Hurler syndrome, but there are treatments that can help to manage the symptoms and improve quality of life. Treatment options include:

Enzyme replacement therapy (ERT): ERT is a treatment that replaces the missing or defective alpha-L-iduronidase enzyme. ERT is given as an infusion into the bloodstream and can help to reduce the buildup of dermatan sulfate in the body.

Gene therapy: Gene therapy is a new treatment that is still in clinical trials. Gene therapy involves replacing the mutated IDUA gene with a healthy copy of the gene. Gene therapy has the potential to cure Hurler syndrome, but it is still too early to say for sure if it will be successful.

Supportive care: Supportive care includes measures such as feeding tube placement, respiratory support, and pain management.

The outlook for people with Hurler syndrome is poor. Most people with Hurler syndrome die in childhood or early adulthood. However, with treatment, people with Hurler syndrome can live longer and have a better quality of life.

If you or your child has been diagnosed with Hurler syndrome, it is important to talk to your doctor about treatment options and how to best manage the disease. There are many resources available to help people with Hurler syndrome and their families, including the Hurler Syndrome Foundation and the MPS Society.

Learn more about Hurler syndrome from the National MPS Society

National MPS Society

PO Box 14686

Durham NC 27709-4686

919.806.0101

Tell me about Sanfilippo syndrome

How was Sanfilippo syndrome discovered?

Sanfilippo syndrome, also known as mucopolysaccharidosis type III (MPS III), is a rare genetic disorder that primarily affects the lysosomal storage of complex carbohydrates. The discovery and understanding of Sanfilippo syndrome involved a series of scientific observations and advancements. Here is an overview of the historical developments in the discovery of Sanfilippo syndrome:

Clinical Observations: In the early 1960s, Dr. Sylvester Sanfilippo, an American pediatrician, described a set of symptoms in children that included developmental delay, progressive neurological deterioration, behavioral problems, and other characteristic features. Dr. Sanfilippo recognized that these cases represented a distinct clinical entity.

Recognition as a Distinct Disorder: Following Dr. Sanfilippo's observations, additional cases with similar features were reported by other physicians, further establishing Sanfilippo syndrome as a distinct disorder. It was classified as a mucopolysaccharidosis, a group of lysosomal storage disorders characterized by the accumulation of complex carbohydrates called mucopolysaccharides.

Biochemical Basis: In the 1970s and 1980s, researchers made significant advancements in understanding the biochemical basis of Sanfilippo syndrome. They discovered that individuals with Sanfilippo syndrome have a deficiency or dysfunction of one of the enzymes involved in the breakdown of heparan sulfate, a specific type of mucopolysaccharide. There are four types of Sanfilippo syndrome, each caused by a deficiency of a specific enzyme: Type A (heparan N-sulfatase), Type B (alpha-N-acetylglucosaminidase), Type C (acetyl-CoA alpha-glucosaminide N-acetyltransferase), and Type D (N-acetylglucosamine 6-sulfatase).

Genetic Discoveries: In the 1990s and early 2000s, the genes associated with Sanfilippo syndrome were identified. Researchers found that mutations in the genes involved in the production of the specific enzymes responsible for heparan sulfate breakdown lead to the enzyme deficiencies in Sanfilippo syndrome. These gene mutations are inherited in an autosomal recessive manner.

Diagnostic Advances: Over time, diagnostic techniques for Sanfilippo syndrome have improved. Measurement of enzyme activity and genetic testing for mutations in the associated genes have become standard diagnostic methods. These tests help confirm the diagnosis, determine the specific subtype of Sanfilippo syndrome, and facilitate genetic counseling and carrier detection.

Treatment Approaches: Currently, there is no cure for Sanfilippo syndrome. Treatment primarily focuses on managing symptoms and providing supportive care. Research is ongoing to explore potential therapies, including enzyme replacement therapy, gene therapy, and substrate reduction therapy, to address the underlying enzyme deficiencies and slow disease progression.

Continued Research: Ongoing research in Sanfilippo syndrome focuses on understanding the disease mechanisms, further improving treatment options, and exploring potential therapeutic approaches. Scientists are investigating various strategies, including gene editing, stem cell transplantation, and novel drug therapies, to target the underlying genetic defects and alleviate the symptoms of Sanfilippo syndrome.

The discovery and ongoing research in Sanfilippo syndrome have led to improved diagnostic techniques, increased understanding of the disease biology, and the exploration of potential treatment options. These efforts contribute to improving the management and quality of life for individuals affected by Sanfilippo syndrome.

What is Sanfilippo syndrome?

Sanfilippo syndrome (also known as mucopolysaccharidosis type III (MPS III)) is a rare, inherited metabolic disorder that affects the body's ability to break down certain complex sugars. This leads to the buildup of these sugars in the body's tissues, which can cause a variety of problems, including intellectual disability, behavioral problems, and physical decline.

Sanfilippo syndrome is caused by a mutation in one of four genes that code for enzymes that break down heparan sulfate. Heparan sulfate is a type of complex sugar that is found throughout the body. When the enzymes that break down heparan sulfate are not working properly, heparan sulfate builds up in the body's tissues.

Sanfilippo syndrome is inherited in an autosomal recessive manner, which means that both parents must carry a mutated gene in order for their child to be born with the disease.

The symptoms of Sanfilippo syndrome can vary from person to person, but they typically begin in early childhood. Common symptoms include:

Intellectual disability: Children with Sanfilippo syndrome typically have intellectual disability that worsens over time.

Behavioral problems: Children with Sanfilippo syndrome may have behavioral problems, such as hyperactivity, aggression, and self-injury.

Physical decline: Children with Sanfilippo syndrome may experience physical decline, such as muscle weakness, joint stiffness, and difficulty walking.

Sleep problems: Children with Sanfilippo syndrome may have sleep problems, such as difficulty falling asleep and staying asleep.

Seizures: Some children with Sanfilippo syndrome may experience seizures.

There is no cure for Sanfilippo syndrome, but there are treatments that can help to manage the symptoms and improve quality of life. Treatment options include:

Enzyme replacement therapy (ERT): ERT is a treatment that replaces the missing or defective enzymes that break down heparan sulfate. ERT is given as an infusion into the bloodstream and can help to reduce the buildup of heparan sulfate in the body.

Gene therapy: Gene therapy is a new treatment that is still in clinical trials. Gene therapy involves replacing the mutated genes that cause Sanfilippo syndrome with healthy copies of the genes. Gene therapy has the potential to cure Sanfilippo syndrome, but it is still too early to say for sure if it will be successful.

Supportive care: Supportive care includes measures such as feeding tube placement, respiratory support, and pain management.

The outlook for people with Sanfilippo syndrome is poor. Most people with Sanfilippo syndrome die in their 20s or 30s. However, with treatment, people with Sanfilippo syndrome can live longer and have a better quality of life.

If you or your child has been diagnosed with Sanfilippo syndrome, it is important to talk to your doctor about treatment options and how to best manage the disease. There are many resources available to help people with Sanfilippo syndrome and their families, such as the Sanfilippo Children's Foundation and the MPS Society.

Here are some additional information about Sanfilippo syndrome:

There are four types of Sanfilippo syndrome, each caused by a mutation in a different gene.

The types of Sanfilippo syndrome are named after the researchers who first described them: Sanfilippo A, Sanfilippo B, Sanfilippo C, and Sanfilippo D.

The symptoms of Sanfilippo syndrome vary depending on the type of Sanfilippo syndrome.

The severity of Sanfilippo syndrome also varies depending on the type of Sanfilippo syndrome.

Sanfilippo syndrome is a progressive disease, which means that the symptoms get worse over time.

There is no cure for Sanfilippo syndrome.

Treatment for Sanfilippo syndrome is aimed at managing the symptoms and improving quality of life.

Learn more about Sanfilippo syndrome from team sanfilippo foundation

TSF Inc.

20 Lakewood Avenue

Ronkonkoma, NY 11779

518-879-6571

Tell me about Morquio syndrome

How was Morquio syndrome discovered?

Morquio syndrome, also known as mucopolysaccharidosis type IV (MPS IV), is a rare genetic disorder that primarily affects the lysosomal storage of complex carbohydrates. The discovery and understanding of Morquio syndrome involved a series of scientific observations and advancements. Here is an overview of the historical developments in the discovery of Morquio syndrome:

Clinical Observations: In the early 20th century, Dr. Luis Morquio, a Uruguayan physician, described a set of symptoms in children that included skeletal abnormalities, short stature, joint laxity, and other characteristic features. Dr. Morquio recognized that these cases represented a distinct clinical entity.

Recognition as a Distinct Disorder: Following Dr. Morquio's observations, additional cases with similar features were reported by other physicians, further establishing Morquio syndrome as a distinct disorder. It was classified as a mucopolysaccharidosis, a group of lysosomal storage disorders characterized by the accumulation of complex carbohydrates called mucopolysaccharides.

Biochemical Basis: In the 1960s and 1970s, researchers made significant advancements in understanding the biochemical basis of Morquio syndrome. They discovered that individuals with Morquio syndrome have a deficiency or dysfunction of the enzymes responsible for breaking down specific mucopolysaccharides called keratan sulfate. There are two subtypes of Morquio syndrome: Type A (deficiency of the enzyme N-acetylgalactosamine-6-sulfatase) and Type B (deficiency of the enzyme beta-galactosidase).

Genetic Discoveries: In the 1990s and early 2000s, the genes associated with Morquio syndrome were identified. Researchers found that mutations in the genes responsible for producing the enzymes involved in keratan sulfate breakdown lead to the enzyme deficiencies in Morquio syndrome. These gene mutations are inherited in an autosomal recessive manner.

Diagnostic Advances: Over time, diagnostic techniques for Morquio syndrome have improved. Measurement of enzyme activity and genetic testing for mutations in the associated genes have become standard diagnostic methods. These tests help confirm the diagnosis, determine the specific subtype of Morquio syndrome, and facilitate genetic counseling and carrier detection.

Treatment Approaches: Currently, there is no cure for Morquio syndrome. Treatment primarily focuses on managing symptoms and providing supportive care. Enzyme replacement therapy has shown promise in treating certain aspects of the disease. It involves regular infusions of synthetic forms of the deficient enzymes to help break down accumulated keratan sulfate. Additional therapies, such as surgical interventions to address skeletal abnormalities and supportive care to manage other symptoms, are also provided.

Continued Research: Ongoing research in Morquio syndrome focuses on understanding the disease mechanisms, further improving treatment options, and exploring potential therapeutic approaches. Scientists are investigating various strategies, including gene therapy, substrate reduction therapy, and advanced enzyme replacement therapies, to target the underlying enzyme deficiencies and slow disease progression.

The discovery and ongoing research in Morquio syndrome have led to improved diagnostic techniques, increased understanding of the disease biology, and the exploration of potential treatment options. These efforts contribute to improving the management and quality of life for individuals affected by Morquio syndrome.

What is Morquio syndrome?

Morquio syndrome, also known as mucopolysaccharidosis type IV (MPS IV), is a rare genetic disorder that affects the body's ability to break down certain complex sugars. This leads to the buildup of these sugars in the body's tissues, which can cause a variety of problems, including short stature, skeletal deformities, heart problems, and breathing problems.

Morquio syndrome is caused by a mutation in the NAGLU gene, which is responsible for producing an enzyme called N-acetylgalactosamine-6-sulfate sulfatase. This enzyme is needed to break down a type of complex sugar called keratan sulfate. When the NAGLU gene is mutated, the body cannot produce enough N-acetylgalactosamine-6-sulfate sulfatase, which leads to the buildup of keratan sulfate in the body.

Morquio syndrome is inherited in an autosomal recessive manner, which means that both parents must carry a mutated gene in order for their child to be born with the disease.

The symptoms of Morquio syndrome can vary from person to person, but they typically begin in early childhood. Common symptoms include:

Short stature: Children with Morquio syndrome are typically very short.

Skeletal deformities: Children with Morquio syndrome may have skeletal deformities, such as a hunchback, a curvature of the spine, and knock-knees.

Heart problems: Children with Morquio syndrome may have heart problems, such as enlarged heart and heart valve problems.

Breathing problems: Children with Morquio syndrome may have breathing problems, such as obstructive sleep apnea and chronic lung disease.

Other problems: Children with Morquio syndrome may also experience other problems, such as hearing loss, vision problems, and joint pain.

There is no cure for Morquio syndrome, but there are treatments that can help to manage the symptoms and improve quality of life. Treatment options include:

Enzyme replacement therapy (ERT): ERT is a treatment that replaces the missing or defective N-acetylgalactosamine-6-sulfate sulfatase enzyme. ERT is given as an infusion into the bloodstream and can help to reduce the buildup of keratan sulfate in the body.

Gene therapy: Gene therapy is a new treatment that is still in clinical trials. Gene therapy involves replacing the mutated NAGLU gene with a healthy copy of the gene. Gene therapy has the potential to cure Morquio syndrome, but it is still too early to say for sure if it will be successful.

Supportive care: Supportive care includes measures such as feeding tube placement, respiratory support, and pain management.

The outlook for people with Morquio syndrome varies depending on the severity of the disease. Some people with Morquio syndrome live into their 30s or 40s, while others die in childhood. However, with treatment, people with Morquio syndrome can live long and productive lives.

If you or your child has been diagnosed with Morquio syndrome, it is important to talk to your doctor about treatment options and how to best manage the disease. There are many resources available to help people with Morquio syndrome and their families, such as the Morquio Foundation and the MPS Society.

Here are some additional information about Morquio syndrome:

There is no cure for Morquio syndrome.

Treatment for Morquio syndrome is aimed at managing the symptoms and improving quality of life.

The average life expectancy for people with Morquio syndrome is 30-40 years.

People with Morquio syndrome may experience a range of physical and intellectual disabilities.

There is a strong support network available for people with Morquio syndrome and their families.

Learn more about Morquio Syndrome from the MPS Society

MPS Society, MPS House,

Repton Place, White Lion Road,

Amersham, Buckinghamshire,

HP7 9LP, United Kingdom

0345 389 9901

Tell me about Maroteaux-Lamy syndrome

How was Maroteaux-Lamy syndrome discovered?

Maroteaux-Lamy syndrome, also known as mucopolysaccharidosis type VI (MPS VI), is a rare genetic disorder that primarily affects the lysosomal storage of complex carbohydrates. The discovery and understanding of Maroteaux-Lamy syndrome involved a series of scientific observations and advancements. Here is an overview of the historical developments in the discovery of Maroteaux-Lamy syndrome:

Clinical Observations: In the 1960s, Dr. Pierre Maroteaux, a French pediatrician, and Dr. Maurice Lamy, a French physician, independently described a set of symptoms in children that included skeletal abnormalities, heart valve problems, and other characteristic features. They recognized that these cases represented a distinct clinical entity.

Recognition as a Distinct Disorder: Following the clinical observations by Maroteaux and Lamy, additional cases with similar features were reported by other physicians, further establishing Maroteaux-Lamy syndrome as a distinct disorder. It was classified as a mucopolysaccharidosis, a group of lysosomal storage disorders characterized by the accumulation of complex carbohydrates called mucopolysaccharides.

Biochemical Basis: In the 1970s and 1980s, researchers made significant advancements in understanding the biochemical basis of Maroteaux-Lamy syndrome. They discovered that individuals with Maroteaux-Lamy syndrome have a deficiency or dysfunction of the enzyme called N-acetylgalactosamine 4-sulfatase (also known as arylsulfatase B). This enzyme is responsible for breaking down a specific mucopolysaccharide called dermatan sulfate.

Genetic Discoveries: In the 1990s and early 2000s, the gene associated with Maroteaux-Lamy syndrome was identified. Researchers found that mutations in the gene responsible for producing the arylsulfatase B enzyme lead to its deficiency in Maroteaux-Lamy syndrome. These gene mutations are inherited in an autosomal recessive manner.

Diagnostic Advances: Over time, diagnostic techniques for Maroteaux-Lamy syndrome have improved. Measurement of enzyme activity and genetic testing for mutations in the associated gene have become standard diagnostic methods. These tests help confirm the diagnosis, determine the specific subtype of Maroteaux-Lamy syndrome, and facilitate genetic counseling and carrier detection.

Treatment Approaches: Currently, there is no cure for Maroteaux-Lamy syndrome. Treatment primarily focuses on managing symptoms and providing supportive care. Enzyme replacement therapy has shown promise in treating certain aspects of the disease. It involves regular infusions of synthetic forms of the deficient arylsulfatase B enzyme to help break down accumulated dermatan sulfate. Additional therapies, such as surgical interventions to address skeletal abnormalities, cardiac care for heart valve problems, and supportive care to manage other symptoms, are also provided.

Continued Research: Ongoing research in Maroteaux-Lamy syndrome focuses on understanding the disease mechanisms, further improving treatment options, and exploring potential therapeutic approaches. Scientists are investigating various strategies, including gene therapy, substrate reduction therapy, and advanced enzyme replacement therapies, to target the underlying enzyme deficiency and slow disease progression.

The discovery and ongoing research in Maroteaux-Lamy syndrome have led to improved diagnostic techniques, increased understanding of the disease biology, and the exploration of potential treatment options. These efforts contribute to improving the management and quality of life for individuals affected by Maroteaux-Lamy syndrome.

What is Maroteaux-Lamy syndrome?

Maroteaux-Lamy syndrome (MPS VI), also known as mucopolysaccharidosis type VI, is a rare genetic disorder that affects the body's ability to break down certain complex sugars. This leads to the buildup of these sugars in the body's tissues, which can cause a variety of problems, including short stature, skeletal deformities, heart problems, and breathing problems.

Maroteaux-Lamy syndrome is caused by a mutation in the ARSB gene, which is responsible for producing an enzyme called arylsulfatase B. This enzyme is needed to break down a type of complex sugar called dermatan sulfate. When the ARSB gene is mutated, the body cannot produce enough arylsulfatase B, which leads to the buildup of dermatan sulfate in the body.

Maroteaux-Lamy syndrome is inherited in an autosomal recessive manner, which means that both parents must carry a mutated gene in order for their child to be born with the disease.

The symptoms of Maroteaux-Lamy syndrome can vary from person to person, but they typically begin in early childhood. Common symptoms include:

Short stature: Children with Maroteaux-Lamy syndrome are typically very short.

Skeletal deformities: Children with Maroteaux-Lamy syndrome may have skeletal deformities, such as a hunchback, a curvature of the spine, and knock-knees.

Heart problems: Children with Maroteaux-Lamy syndrome may have heart problems, such as enlarged heart and heart valve problems.

Breathing problems: Children with Maroteaux-Lamy syndrome may have breathing problems, such as obstructive sleep apnea and chronic lung disease.

Other problems: Children with Maroteaux-Lamy syndrome may also experience other problems, such as hearing loss, vision problems, and joint pain.

There is no cure for Maroteaux-Lamy syndrome, but there are treatments that can help to manage the symptoms and improve quality of life. Treatment options include:

Enzyme replacement therapy (ERT): ERT is a treatment that replaces the missing or defective arylsulfatase B enzyme. ERT is given as an infusion into the bloodstream and can help to reduce the buildup of dermatan sulfate in the body.

Gene therapy: Gene therapy is a new treatment that is still in clinical trials. Gene therapy involves replacing the mutated ARSB gene with a healthy copy of the gene. Gene therapy has the potential to cure Maroteaux-Lamy syndrome, but it is still too early to say for sure if it will be successful.

Supportive care: Supportive care includes measures such as feeding tube placement, respiratory support, and pain management.

The outlook for people with Maroteaux-Lamy syndrome varies depending on the severity of the disease. Some people with Maroteaux-Lamy syndrome live into their 30s or 40s, while others die in childhood. However, with treatment, people with Maroteaux-Lamy syndrome can live long and productive lives.

If you or your child has been diagnosed with Maroteaux-Lamy syndrome, it is important to talk to your doctor about treatment options and how to best manage the disease. There are many resources available to help people with Maroteaux-Lamy syndrome and their families, such as the Maroteaux-Lamy Foundation and the MPS Society.

Here are some additional information about Maroteaux-Lamy syndrome:

There is no cure for Maroteaux-Lamy syndrome.

Treatment for Maroteaux-Lamy syndrome is aimed at managing the symptoms and improving quality of life.

The average life expectancy for people with Maroteaux-Lamy syndrome is 30-40 years.

People with Maroteaux-Lamy syndrome may experience a range of physical and intellectual disabilities.

There is a strong support network available for people with Maroteaux-Lamy syndrome and their families.

Learn more about Maroteaux-Lamy syndrome from the MPS Society

National MPS Society

PO Box 14686

Durham NC 27709-4686

919.806.0101

Tell me about Adrenoleukodystrophy

How was Adrenoleukodystrophy discovered?

Adrenoleukodystrophy (ALD) was discovered through a combination of clinical observations, biochemical investigations, and genetic research. Here is an overview of the discovery of Adrenoleukodystrophy:

Clinical Observations: Adrenoleukodystrophy was first recognized and described by Dr. Siemerling and Dr. Creutzfeldt in 1923. They observed a set of symptoms in boys, including adrenal insufficiency (failure of the adrenal glands to produce certain hormones), neurological deterioration, and demyelination (loss of the protective myelin sheath surrounding nerve cells). These observations formed the initial clinical understanding of the disease.

Identification of Peroxisomal Dysfunction: In the 1960s, further investigations revealed that Adrenoleukodystrophy involved a dysfunction of peroxisomes, specialized cellular structures involved in various metabolic processes. Researchers found that peroxisomal fatty acid oxidation was impaired in individuals with Adrenoleukodystrophy, leading to the accumulation of very-long-chain fatty acids (VLCFAs) in various tissues.

Biochemical Studies: In the 1980s, researchers conducted biochemical studies to understand the underlying metabolic abnormalities in Adrenoleukodystrophy. They found significantly elevated levels of VLCFAs, particularly in the blood plasma and adrenal cortex, confirming the metabolic disturbance associated with the disease.

Genetic Discoveries: In the late 1980s and early 1990s, the gene responsible for Adrenoleukodystrophy was identified. Researchers found that mutations in the ABCD1 gene located on the X chromosome are responsible for the disease. These gene mutations lead to a deficiency or dysfunction of a specific protein called ALD protein or ABCD1 protein, which is involved in the transport of VLCFAs into peroxisomes.

Diagnostic Advances: With the identification of the ABCD1 gene, genetic testing became a valuable tool for diagnosing Adrenoleukodystrophy. Testing for mutations in the ABCD1 gene helps confirm the diagnosis, determine the specific subtype of Adrenoleukodystrophy, and facilitate genetic counseling and carrier detection. Additionally, measurement of VLCFAs in blood samples can aid in the diagnosis of the condition.

Treatment Approaches: The treatment of Adrenoleukodystrophy depends on the subtype and stage of the disease. Hematopoietic stem cell transplantation (HSCT) has been effective in halting the progression of the disease in certain individuals when performed early in the course of cerebral involvement. Newer therapies, such as gene therapy and pharmacological approaches, are also being investigated for their potential to treat Adrenoleukodystrophy.

Continued Research: Ongoing research in Adrenoleukodystrophy focuses on further understanding the disease mechanisms, developing improved diagnostic techniques, and exploring novel treatment options. Scientists are investigating the role of VLCFAs in disease progression, exploring potential therapeutic targets, and conducting clinical trials to evaluate the efficacy of various treatment strategies.

The discovery and ongoing research in Adrenoleukodystrophy have contributed to improved diagnostic methods, increased understanding of the disease biology, and the development of treatment options. These advancements have improved the management and outcomes for individuals affected by Adrenoleukodystrophy.

What is Adrenoleukodystrophy?

Adrenoleukodystrophy (ALD) is a rare genetic disorder that affects the body's ability to break down very long chain fatty acids (VLCFAs). This leads to the buildup of VLCFAs in the brain, spinal cord, and adrenal glands. The buildup of VLCFAs damages the myelin sheath, which is a fatty substance that insulates nerve cells. This damage can lead to a variety of problems, including neurological problems, vision problems, and adrenal insufficiency.

ALD is caused by a mutation in the ABCD1 gene, which is responsible for producing an enzyme called adrenoleukodystrophy protein (ALDP). ALDP is needed to break down VLCFAs. When the ABCD1 gene is mutated, the body cannot produce enough ALDP, which leads to the buildup of VLCFAs in the body.

ALD is inherited in an X-linked recessive manner, which means that a boy only needs to inherit one mutated copy of the ABCD1 gene from his mother in order to be born with the disease. Girls who inherit one mutated copy of the ABCD1 gene are carriers, but they do not typically show any symptoms of the disease.

The symptoms of ALD can vary from person to person, but they typically begin in early childhood. Common symptoms include:

Behavioral changes: Children with ALD may experience behavioral changes, such as irritability, aggression, and mood swings.

Vision problems: Children with ALD may experience vision problems, such as double vision, loss of peripheral vision, and vision loss.

Adrenal insufficiency: Children with ALD may experience adrenal insufficiency, which is a condition in which the adrenal glands do not produce enough hormones. Symptoms of adrenal insufficiency can include fatigue, weakness, weight loss, and low blood pressure.

Other problems: Children with ALD may also experience other problems, such as seizures, hearing loss, and difficulty walking.

There is no cure for ALD, but there are treatments that can help to manage the symptoms and improve quality of life. Treatment options include:

Enzyme replacement therapy (ERT): ERT is a treatment that replaces the missing or defective ALDP enzyme. ERT is given as an infusion into the bloodstream and can help to reduce the buildup of VLCFAs in the body.

Gene therapy: Gene therapy is a new treatment that is still in clinical trials. Gene therapy involves replacing the mutated ABCD1 gene with a healthy copy of the gene. Gene therapy has the potential to cure ALD, but it is still too early to say for sure if it will be successful.

Supportive care: Supportive care includes measures such as feeding tube placement, respiratory support, and pain management.

The outlook for people with ALD varies depending on the severity of the disease. Some people with ALD live into their 20s or 30s, while others die in childhood. However, with treatment, people with ALD can live long and productive lives.

If you or your child has been diagnosed with ALD, it is important to talk to your doctor about treatment options and how to best manage the disease. There are many resources available to help people with ALD and their families, such as the ALD Foundation and the National Organization for Rare Disorders (NORD).

Learn more about Andrenoleukodystrophy from ALD Connect

ALD Connect

35 Village Road Suite 100 #353306

Middleton, MA 01949

(833) 525-3266

Tell me about Metachromatic leukodystrophy

How was Metachromatic leukodystrophy discovered?

Metachromatic leukodystrophy (MLD) was discovered through a combination of clinical observations, histopathological studies, and biochemical investigations. Here is an overview of the discovery of Metachromatic leukodystrophy:

Clinical Observations: The clinical features of Metachromatic leukodystrophy were first described by a German neurologist named Dr. Ernst Siemerling in 1923. He observed a group of patients who exhibited progressive neurological deterioration, loss of motor skills, and changes in behavior and cognition. These observations formed the initial clinical understanding of the disease.

Histopathological Studies: In the 1930s, Dr. Marianne Wolff, a German neuropathologist, conducted histopathological examinations of the brains of individuals with Metachromatic leukodystrophy. She observed abnormal accumulations of a substance called metachromatic material in the brain tissue. This metachromatic material stained differently when exposed to certain dyes, revealing characteristic cellular changes that helped differentiate MLD from other disorders.

Biochemical Studies: In the 1950s and 1960s, researchers conducted biochemical investigations to understand the underlying metabolic abnormalities in Metachromatic leukodystrophy. They found that the metachromatic material accumulating in the brain and other tissues was composed of a specific lipid called sulfatide. Further studies showed that individuals with MLD had a deficiency of the enzyme arylsulfatase A, which is responsible for breaking down sulfatides.

Genetic Discoveries: In the 1980s, the gene associated with Metachromatic leukodystrophy was identified. Researchers found that mutations in the ARSA gene, which encodes the arylsulfatase A enzyme, lead to the deficiency of this enzyme and the subsequent accumulation of sulfatides. These gene mutations are inherited in an autosomal recessive manner.

Diagnostic Advances: With the identification of the ARSA gene mutations, genetic testing became a valuable tool for diagnosing Metachromatic leukodystrophy. Testing for mutations in the ARSA gene helps confirm the diagnosis, determine the specific subtype of MLD, and facilitate genetic counseling and carrier detection. Measurement of arylsulfatase A enzyme

activity and analysis of sulfatide levels in urine and blood samples can also aid in the diagnosis of the condition.

Treatment Approaches: Currently, there is no cure for Metachromatic leukodystrophy, and treatment focuses on managing symptoms and providing supportive care. Hematopoietic stem cell transplantation (HSCT) has shown some benefit in individuals with early-onset MLD. Experimental approaches, such as enzyme replacement therapy and gene therapy, are being investigated for their potential to treat the disease.

Continued Research: Ongoing research in Metachromatic leukodystrophy aims to further understand the disease mechanisms, develop improved diagnostic techniques, and explore novel treatment strategies. Scientists are studying the role of sulfatide accumulation in disease progression, investigating potential therapeutic targets, and conducting clinical trials to assess the efficacy of different treatment approaches.

The discovery and ongoing research in Metachromatic leukodystrophy have led to a better understanding of the disease, improved diagnostic methods, and the development of potential treatment options. These advancements contribute to enhanced care and management for individuals affected by Metachromatic leukodystrophy.

What is Metachromatic leukodystrophy?

Metachromatic leukodystrophy (MLD) is a rare genetic disorder that affects the body's ability to break down a type of fat called sulfatide. This leads to the buildup of sulfatide in the brain and spinal cord, which can damage the myelin sheath, a fatty substance that insulates nerve cells. This damage can lead to a variety of problems, including neurological problems, vision problems, and hearing loss.

MLD is caused by a mutation in the ARSA gene, which is responsible for producing an enzyme called arylsulfatase A. ARSA is needed to break down sulfatide. When the ARSA gene is mutated, the body cannot produce enough ARSA, which leads to the buildup of sulfatide in the body.

MLD is inherited in an autosomal recessive manner, which means that both parents must carry a mutated copy of the ARSA gene in order for their child to be born with the disease.

The symptoms of MLD can vary from person to person, but they typically begin in early childhood. Common symptoms include:

Behavioral changes: Children with MLD may experience behavioral changes, such as irritability, aggression, and mood swings.

Vision problems: Children with MLD may experience vision problems, such as double vision, loss of peripheral vision, and vision loss.

Hearing loss: Children with MLD may experience hearing loss.

Other problems: Children with MLD may also experience other problems, such as seizures, difficulty walking, and intellectual disability.

There is no cure for MLD, but there are treatments that can help to manage the symptoms and improve quality of life. Treatment options include:

Enzyme replacement therapy (ERT): ERT is a treatment that replaces the missing or defective ARSA enzyme. ERT is given as an infusion into the bloodstream and can help to reduce the buildup of sulfatide in the body.

Gene therapy: Gene therapy is a new treatment that is still in clinical trials. Gene therapy involves replacing the mutated ARSA gene with a healthy copy of the gene. Gene therapy has the potential to cure MLD, but it is still too early to say for sure if it will be successful.

Supportive care: Supportive care includes measures such as feeding tube placement, respiratory support, and pain management.

The outlook for people with MLD varies depending on the severity of the disease. Some people with MLD live into their 20s or 30s, while others die in childhood. However, with treatment, people with MLD can live long and productive lives.

If you or your child has been diagnosed with MLD, it is important to talk to your doctor about treatment options and how to best manage the disease. There are many resources available to help people with MLD and their families, such as the Metachromatic Leukodystrophy Association (MLA) and the National Organization for Rare Disorders (NORD).

Learn more about Metachromatic leukodystrophy from the MLD foundation

Tell me about Canavan disease

How was Canavan disease discovered?

Canavan disease was discovered through a combination of clinical observations, histopathological studies, and genetic investigations. Here is an overview of the discovery of Canavan disease:

Clinical Observations: Canavan disease was first described by a Swiss-American pediatrician named Myrtelle Canavan in 1931. She observed a group of infants who displayed severe neurological symptoms, including progressive developmental delays, abnormal muscle tone, and impaired head control. These observations formed the initial clinical understanding of the disease.

Histopathological Studies: In the 1960s, further investigations were conducted to study the brain pathology in individuals with Canavan disease. Histopathological studies revealed significant abnormalities in the white matter of the brain, particularly the loss of myelin, which is the protective covering around nerve fibers. This led to the recognition of Canavan disease as a leukodystrophy, a group of disorders characterized by abnormalities in the production or maintenance of myelin.

Biochemical Studies: In the 1980s, researchers conducted biochemical investigations to understand the underlying metabolic abnormalities in Canavan disease. They found that affected individuals had significantly increased levels of a substance called N-acetyl-L-aspartic acid (NAA) in their urine, blood, and cerebrospinal fluid. This abnormal accumulation of NAA became a key diagnostic marker for Canavan disease.

Genetic Discoveries: In the 1990s, the gene responsible for Canavan disease was identified. Researchers found that mutations in the ASPA gene, which encodes an enzyme called aspartoacylase, lead to the accumulation of NAA in the brain and subsequent destruction of myelin. These gene mutations are inherited in an autosomal recessive manner.

Diagnostic Advances: With the identification of the ASPA gene mutations, genetic testing became a valuable tool for diagnosing Canavan disease. Testing for mutations in the ASPA gene helps confirm the diagnosis, determine the specific subtype of Canavan disease, and facilitate genetic counseling and carrier detection. Measurement of NAA levels in urine, blood, or cerebrospinal fluid can also aid in the diagnosis of the condition.

Treatment Approaches: Currently, there is no cure for Canavan disease, and treatment focuses on managing symptoms and providing supportive care. Various therapeutic approaches, including dietary modifications, physical therapy, and medication, are utilized to address specific symptoms and improve quality of life for affected individuals.

Continued Research: Ongoing research in Canavan disease aims to further understand the disease mechanisms, develop improved diagnostic methods, and explore potential treatment strategies. Scientists are studying the role of aspartoacylase enzyme deficiency in disease progression, investigating potential therapeutic targets, and exploring experimental approaches such as gene therapy.

The discovery and ongoing research in Canavan disease have contributed to a better understanding of the disease, improved diagnostic methods, and the development of supportive care strategies. These advancements enhance the management and quality of life for individuals affected by Canavan disease.

What is Canavan disease?

Canavan disease is a rare, inherited disorder that affects the nervous system. It is caused by a mutation in the gene that codes for the enzyme aspartoacylase, which breaks down a substance called N-acetylaspartic acid (NAA). When this enzyme is missing or defective, NAA builds up in the brain and spinal cord, causing damage to nerve cells.

Canavan disease is inherited in an autosomal recessive manner, which means that both parents must carry a mutated copy of the gene in order for their child to be born with the disease.

The symptoms of Canavan disease usually begin in early infancy. Affected infants may have difficulty feeding, poor muscle tone, and seizures. As the disease progresses, children with Canavan disease may experience intellectual disability, vision problems, hearing loss, and difficulty walking. Death typically occurs in childhood or early adulthood.

There is no cure for Canavan disease. Treatment is supportive and aimed at managing the symptoms. Treatment options may include:

Diet: Children with Canavan disease may need to be fed a special diet that is low in NAA.

Seizure control: Medications may be used to control seizures.

Physical therapy: Physical therapy can help to improve muscle tone and movement.

Speech therapy: Speech therapy can help to improve communication skills.

Other supportive care: Other supportive care measures may include feeding tube placement, respiratory support, and pain management.

Canavan disease is a serious and life-limiting condition. However, with early diagnosis and treatment, children with Canavan disease can live long and fulfilling lives.

If you or your child has been diagnosed with Canavan disease, it is important to talk to your doctor about treatment options and how to best manage the disease. There are many resources available to help people with Canavan disease and their families, such as the Canavan Foundation and the National Organization for Rare Disorders (NORD).

Learn more about Canavan disease from the Canavan Project

Tell me about Alexander disease

How was Alexander disease discovered?

Alexander disease was first discovered and described by two researchers, William Stewart Alexander and his colleague Ronald W. Leech, in 1949. They published their findings in the journal Brain, titled "Diffuse Progressive Degeneration of the Gray Matter of the Cerebral Hemispheres in Infancy."

The discovery of Alexander disease came about through the examination and analysis of brain tissue from affected individuals. Alexander and Leech conducted autopsies on several children who had exhibited severe neurological symptoms and progressive degeneration of the brain. They observed distinct pathological features, including the presence of abnormal structures known as Rosenthal fibers. These Rosenthal fibers, composed of a protein called glial fibrillary acidic protein (GFAP), were found throughout the brain tissue, particularly in the white matter and astrocytes.

Based on their observations, Alexander and Leech proposed that the accumulation of Rosenthal fibers in the brain tissue was indicative of a distinct neurodegenerative disorder, which they named Alexander disease in honor of Dr. William Stewart Alexander.

Since the initial discovery, further research has been conducted to better understand the underlying genetic and molecular basis of Alexander disease. It has been found that mutations in the GFAP gene are responsible for the majority of cases of Alexander disease. These mutations lead to abnormal aggregation and accumulation of GFAP, resulting in the formation of Rosenthal fibers and the subsequent damage to astrocytes.

Subsequent studies have expanded the knowledge of Alexander disease, including its different subtypes and associated clinical manifestations. Advances in genetic testing and diagnostic techniques have facilitated the identification of GFAP gene mutations and improved the accuracy of diagnosis.

Ongoing research continues to explore the underlying mechanisms of Alexander disease, including the role of GFAP and astrocyte dysfunction in disease progression. Experimental approaches, such as gene therapy and targeted treatments, are being investigated to develop potential therapies for this rare and devastating neurological disorder.

What is Alexander disease?

Alexander disease is a rare, genetic disorder that affects the brain and spinal cord. It is caused by a mutation in the GFAP gene, which codes for the protein glial fibrillary acidic protein (GFAP). GFAP is a structural protein that helps to support and protect nerve cells. When the GFAP gene is mutated, GFAP is not produced or is produced abnormally, which can lead to the buildup of abnormal protein clumps called Rosenthal fibers in the brain and spinal cord. These Rosenthal fibers can damage nerve cells and lead to a variety of neurological problems.

Alexander disease is inherited in an autosomal dominant manner, which means that only one mutated copy of the GFAP gene is needed for a person to develop the disease. However, not everyone who inherits a mutated GFAP gene will develop Alexander disease. The risk of developing Alexander disease is higher if the mutated GFAP gene is inherited from a parent who has the disease.

The symptoms of Alexander disease can vary from person to person, but they typically begin in early childhood. Common symptoms include:

Enlarged head (macrocephaly)

Seizures

Intellectual disability

Stiffness of the muscles (spasticity)

Vision problems

Hearing loss

Difficulty walking

Failure to thrive

The prognosis for people with Alexander disease is variable. Some people with Alexander disease live into adulthood, while others die in childhood. There is no cure for Alexander disease, but there are treatments that can help to manage the symptoms and improve quality of life. Treatment options may include:

Seizure control: Medications may be used to control seizures.

Physical therapy: Physical therapy can help to improve muscle tone and movement.

Speech therapy: Speech therapy can help to improve communication skills.

Other supportive care: Other supportive care measures may include feeding tube placement, respiratory support, and pain management.

If you or your child has been diagnosed with Alexander disease, it is important to talk to your doctor about treatment options and how to best manage the disease. There are many resources available to help people with Alexander disease and their families, such as the Alexander Disease Foundation and the National Organization for Rare Disorders (NORD).

Learn more about Alexander disease from the United Leukodystrophy Foundation

ULF

224 North Second Street, Suite 2

DeKalb, IL 60115, USA

+1 (815) 748-0844

Tell me about Pelizaeus-Merzbacher disease

How was Pelizaeus-Merzbacher disease discovered?

Pelizaeus-Merzbacher disease (PMD) was first described by two physicians, Friedrich Pelizaeus and Ludwig Merzbacher, in the early 20th century. They independently made separate observations and contributions to the understanding of the disease. Here is an overview of how Pelizaeus-Merzbacher disease was discovered:

Friedrich Pelizaeus: In 1885, Friedrich Pelizaeus, a German neurologist, described a case of a young boy who presented with nystagmus (involuntary eye movement), spasticity (stiffness and increased muscle tone), and other neurological symptoms. Pelizaeus recognized that the boy's symptoms were distinct from other known conditions and characterized the disorder as a distinct clinical entity.

Ludwig Merzbacher: In 1910, Ludwig Merzbacher, another German physician and neuropathologist, published a detailed case report of two brothers who displayed similar neurological symptoms. Merzbacher performed autopsies on the brothers and conducted histological examinations of their brain tissues. He observed significant abnormalities in the white matter of the brain, particularly in the formation and maintenance of myelin, the protective covering around nerve fibers. Merzbacher recognized that the disorder affected the central nervous system and proposed the term "cerebral sclerosis en plaque" to describe the disease.

Consolidation and Refinement: Over time, the observations and findings of Pelizaeus and Merzbacher were recognized as representing the same disorder. The term "Pelizaeus-Merzbacher disease" was coined to honor both physicians for their contributions. The characteristic features of PMD, including nystagmus, spasticity, and abnormalities in myelin formation, became well-established.

Genetic Discoveries: Subsequent research in the 1990s and early 2000s identified mutations in the PLP1 gene (proteolipid protein 1) as the underlying cause of Pelizaeus-Merzbacher disease. These mutations affect the production or structure of myelin proteins, leading to abnormal myelination in the central nervous system. Pelizaeus-Merzbacher disease is inherited in an X-linked pattern, meaning it primarily affects males.

Diagnostic Advances: The identification of PLP1 gene mutations has facilitated the development of genetic testing methods for diagnosing Pelizaeus-Merzbacher disease.

Genetic testing allows for confirmation of the diagnosis, determination of the specific subtype of PMD, and genetic counseling for affected families. Additional diagnostic techniques, such as brain imaging (MRI), can aid in assessing the extent of white matter abnormalities.

Continued Research: Ongoing research in Pelizaeus-Merzbacher disease focuses on further understanding the underlying mechanisms of myelin formation and maintenance, exploring potential therapeutic strategies to address the disease at a molecular level, and investigating novel approaches such as gene therapy.

The discovery and ongoing research in Pelizaeus-Merzbacher disease have led to a better understanding of the disorder, improved diagnostic methods, and potential avenues for future treatments. These advancements contribute to enhanced care and management for individuals affected by Pelizaeus-Merzbacher disease.

What is Pelizaeus-Merzbacher disease?

Pelizaeus-Merzbacher disease (PMD) is a rare, inherited disorder that affects the central nervous system (CNS). It is caused by a mutation in the PLP1 gene, which codes for a protein called proteolipid protein-1 (PLP1). PLP1 is a major component of myelin, the fatty sheath that insulates nerve cells. When the PLP1 gene is mutated, PLP1 is not produced or is produced abnormally, which can lead to a breakdown of myelin in the CNS. This breakdown of myelin can cause a variety of neurological problems, including:

Seizures

Intellectual disability

Stiffness of the muscles (spasticity)

Vision problems

Hearing loss

Difficulty walking

Failure to thrive

The severity of PMD can vary widely, even among people with the same mutation in the PLP1 gene. Some people with PMD may have mild symptoms and live relatively normal lives, while others may have severe symptoms and die in childhood.

There is no cure for PMD, but there are treatments that can help to manage the symptoms and improve quality of life. Treatment options may include:

Seizure control: Medications may be used to control seizures.

Physical therapy: Physical therapy can help to improve muscle tone and movement.

Speech therapy: Speech therapy can help to improve communication skills.

Other supportive care: Other supportive care measures may include feeding tube placement, respiratory support, and pain management.

If you or your child has been diagnosed with PMD, it is important to talk to your doctor about treatment options and how to best manage the disease. There are many resources available to help people with PMD and their families, such as the Pelizaeus-Merzbacher Disease Association and the National Organization for Rare Disorders (NORD).

PMD is a progressive disease, which means that the symptoms will get worse over time. However, with early diagnosis and treatment, people with PMD can live long and fulfilling lives.

Learn more about Pelizaeus-Merzbacher disease from the PMD Foundation

PMD Foundation

P.O. Box 1077

Madison, NJ 07940

1-254-313-9107

Tell me about Ataxia telangiectasia

How was Ataxia telangiectasia discovered?

Ataxia telangiectasia (A-T) was discovered through the collaborative efforts of several researchers and clinicians. Here is an overview of how A-T was discovered:

Initial Observations: In the late 1950s and early 1960s, two separate groups of researchers, led by Syllaba and Henner, independently described a group of children who displayed a combination of neurological symptoms, including ataxia (lack of muscle coordination) and telangiectasias (small dilated blood vessels on the skin and eyes). These initial observations recognized the distinct clinical features of the condition.

Consolidation of Findings: In 1963, an American physician named Louis-Bar, who had previously studied a similar disorder, recognized the similarities between the cases described by Syllaba, Henner, and others. He consolidated the clinical observations and proposed the term "ataxia telangiectasia" to describe the disorder.

Genetic Link: In the 1980s, the genetic basis of A-T was discovered. Researchers identified mutations in the ATM (ataxia telangiectasia mutated) gene as the underlying cause of the condition. The ATM gene is involved in DNA repair and maintenance of genomic stability. Mutations in this gene lead to defective DNA repair mechanisms, which contribute to the cellular and systemic abnormalities seen in A-T.

Identification of the ATM Gene: In 1995, the ATM gene was cloned and characterized. This breakthrough allowed for more precise genetic testing and diagnosis of A-T. It also provided insights into the molecular mechanisms underlying the disease.

Diagnostic Advances: The identification of ATM gene mutations has led to the development of genetic testing methods for diagnosing A-T. Genetic testing can confirm the diagnosis, determine carrier status, and provide genetic counseling for affected families. Additionally, laboratory tests can measure the levels of specific biomarkers, such as alpha-fetoprotein (AFP), which is often elevated in individuals with A-T.

Research and Treatment: Ongoing research in A-T aims to better understand the disease mechanisms, develop targeted therapies to address specific symptoms, and explore potential interventions to improve the quality of life for affected individuals. Treatments currently focus on managing symptoms and providing supportive care, including physical therapy, occupational therapy, and respiratory support.

The discovery of A-T and subsequent research have contributed to a deeper understanding of the disorder, improved diagnostic capabilities, and potential avenues for therapeutic interventions. These advancements enhance the care and management of individuals affected by Ataxia telangiectasia.

What is Ataxia telangiectasia?

Ataxia-telangiectasia (AT) is a rare, inherited disorder that affects the nervous system, immune system, and other body systems. It is caused by a mutation in the ATM gene, which codes for a protein called ATM. ATM is a tumor suppressor gene, which means that it helps to prevent cells from becoming cancerous. When the ATM gene is mutated, cells are more likely to become cancerous.

AT is inherited in an autosomal recessive manner, which means that both parents must carry a mutated copy of the ATM gene in order for their child to be born with the disease.

The symptoms of AT can vary from person to person, but they typically begin in early childhood. Common symptoms include:

Ataxia: Ataxia is a loss of balance and coordination. People with AT may have difficulty walking, running, and using their hands.

Telangiectasias: Telangiectasias are small, dilated blood vessels that are visible on the skin. They are most commonly found on the face, eyelids, ears, and hands.

Immune deficiency: People with AT have a weakened immune system. They are more likely to get infections, such as pneumonia, meningitis, and lymphoma.

Cancer: People with AT have an increased risk of developing cancer, especially leukemia, lymphoma, and breast cancer.

There is no cure for AT. Treatment is supportive and aimed at managing the symptoms. Treatment options may include:

Physical therapy: Physical therapy can help to improve balance and coordination.

Speech therapy: Speech therapy can help to improve communication skills.

Immunotherapy: Immunotherapy is a treatment that helps to boost the immune system. It may be used to treat infections or to prevent cancer.

Cancer treatment: Cancer treatment may be used to treat cancer that develops in people with AT.

AT is a progressive disease, which means that the symptoms will get worse over time. However, with early diagnosis and treatment, people with AT can live long and fulfilling lives.

If you or your child has been diagnosed with AT, it is important to talk to your doctor about treatment options and how to best manage the disease. There are many resources available to help people with AT and their families, such as the Ataxia-Telangiectasia Association and the National Organization for Rare Disorders (NORD).

Learn more about Ataxia telangiectasia from the AT Children's Project

AT Children's Project

6810 N. State Road 7, Suite 125

Coconut Creek, FL 33073 USA

800.543.5728

Tell me about Fanconi anemia

How was Fanconi anemia discovered?

Fanconi anemia (FA) was discovered through the collaborative efforts of several researchers and clinicians. Here is an overview of how FA was discovered:

Observations and Characterization: In 1927, the Swiss pediatrician Guido Fanconi described a group of children who presented with a combination of physical abnormalities, bone marrow failure, and a predisposition to cancer. He recognized that these cases represented a distinct clinical entity and coined the term "Fanconi anemia."

Genetic Component: In the 1960s, further studies by geneticists and hematologists indicated that Fanconi anemia had a genetic basis. Researchers observed that the condition tended to run in families and showed autosomal recessive inheritance, meaning it required the presence of two mutated genes, one from each parent, for the disease to manifest.

Chromosomal Abnormalities: In the 1980s, cytogenetic studies revealed chromosomal abnormalities in individuals with FA. Researchers discovered that when exposed to certain chemicals or DNA-damaging agents, the cells of individuals with FA exhibited increased chromosomal breakage and rearrangements.

Discovery of FANC Genes: In the late 1990s and early 2000s, the identification of specific genes associated with Fanconi anemia occurred. Researchers found that mutations in at least 23 different genes, now known as the FANC genes, could cause various subtypes of FA. These genes play crucial roles in DNA repair and maintenance of genomic stability.

Functional Understanding: Over time, research has focused on understanding the precise functions of the FANC genes and how their dysfunction contributes to the characteristic features of FA. The FANC genes are involved in DNA repair pathways, particularly the repair of DNA interstrand crosslinks, which are abnormal links between the two strands of DNA.

Diagnostic Advances: The discovery of the FANC genes has facilitated the development of genetic testing methods for diagnosing Fanconi anemia. Genetic testing can identify mutations in the FANC genes, confirm the diagnosis, determine the subtype of FA, and provide genetic counseling for affected families. Additionally, laboratory tests, such as chromosomal breakage analysis, can help support the diagnosis of FA.

Research and Treatment: Ongoing research in Fanconi anemia aims to deepen the understanding of the disease mechanisms, explore potential therapeutic strategies, and develop treatments that address the underlying genetic and cellular defects. Hematopoietic stem cell transplantation is currently the primary treatment option for FA, although gene therapy and other experimental approaches are being investigated.

The discovery of Fanconi anemia and subsequent research have contributed to improved diagnostic methods, a better understanding of the disease's genetic basis and cellular mechanisms, and the development of interventions that enhance the care and management of individuals with Fanconi anemia.

What is Fanconi anemia?

Fanconi anemia (FA) is a rare genetic disorder that affects the bone marrow. It is characterized by a decrease in the production of all types of blood cells, including red blood cells, white blood cells, and platelets. This can lead to a variety of health problems, including anemia, infections, and bleeding disorders.

FA is caused by mutations in one of 22 genes that are involved in DNA repair. These mutations lead to a defect in the way that cells repair damage to their DNA. This can lead to the accumulation of mutations in the bone marrow cells, which eventually leads to their failure to function properly.

FA is inherited in an autosomal recessive manner, which means that both parents must carry a mutated copy of the gene in order for their child to be born with the disease.

The symptoms of FA can vary from person to person, but they typically begin in childhood. Common symptoms include:

Anemia: Anemia is a condition in which the body does not have enough red blood cells. This can lead to fatigue, shortness of breath, and pale skin.

Infections: People with FA have a weakened immune system. They are more likely to get infections, such as pneumonia, meningitis, and sepsis.

Bleeding disorders: People with FA have a tendency to bleed easily. This can be due to a decrease in the number of platelets, which are cells that help to clot blood.

Other symptoms: People with FA may also experience other symptoms, such as:

Short stature

Skin abnormalities, such as café au lait spots and vitiligo

Heart defects

Kidney problems

Increased risk of cancer

There is no cure for FA. Treatment is aimed at managing the symptoms and preventing complications. Treatment options may include:

Blood transfusions: Blood transfusions are used to treat anemia and to prevent bleeding.

Antibiotics: Antibiotics are used to treat infections.

Growth hormone therapy: Growth hormone therapy can help to improve growth and development.

Bone marrow transplantation: Bone marrow transplantation is a procedure in which healthy bone marrow cells are transplanted into the body. This can be a cure for FA, but it is a risky procedure.

The outlook for people with FA varies depending on the severity of the disease. Some people with FA live long and healthy lives, while others die in childhood.

If you or your child has been diagnosed with FA, it is important to talk to your doctor about treatment options and how to best manage the disease. There are many resources available to help people with FA and their families, such as the Fanconi Anemia Research Fund and the National Organization for Rare Disorders (NORD).

Learn more about Fanconi anemia from the Fanconi Anemia Research Fund

Fanconi Anemia Research Fund

360 E. 10th Ave., Suite 201

Eugene, OR 97401

1-888-326-2664

1-541-687-4658

Tell me about Wiskott-Aldrich syndrome

How was Wiskott-Aldrich syndrome discovered?

Wiskott-Aldrich syndrome (WAS) was discovered through the collaborative efforts of several researchers and clinicians. Here is an overview of how WAS was discovered:

Initial Observations: In the late 1930s, two separate physicians, Dr. Alfred Wiskott in Germany and Dr. Robert Aldrich in the United States, independently described a group of male children who presented with recurrent infections, eczema (skin inflammation), and a bleeding tendency. They recognized the distinct clinical features of the condition and reported their findings.

Consolidation of Findings: In 1954, Dr. Robert Good, an American immunologist, reviewed the cases described by Wiskott and Aldrich and recognized the similarities. He consolidated the clinical observations and proposed the term "Wiskott-Aldrich syndrome" to describe the disorder.

Genetic Link: In the 1990s, the genetic basis of Wiskott-Aldrich syndrome was discovered. Researchers identified mutations in the gene encoding the Wiskott-Aldrich syndrome protein (WASP) as the underlying cause of the condition. The WASP gene is responsible for regulating the cytoskeleton, which is essential for various cellular processes, including immune cell function and platelet production.

Identification of the WASP Gene: In 1994, the WASP gene was cloned and characterized. This breakthrough allowed for more precise genetic testing and diagnosis of Wiskott-Aldrich syndrome. It also provided insights into the molecular mechanisms underlying the disease.

Diagnostic Advances: The identification of WASP gene mutations has led to the development of genetic testing methods for diagnosing Wiskott-Aldrich syndrome. Genetic testing can confirm the diagnosis, determine carrier status, and provide genetic counseling for affected families. Additionally, laboratory tests can evaluate immune cell function and platelet parameters to support the diagnosis of WAS.

Research and Treatment: Ongoing research in Wiskott-Aldrich syndrome focuses on further understanding the disease mechanisms, exploring potential therapeutic strategies, and developing interventions to address specific symptoms. Treatment options for Wiskott-Aldrich syndrome include supportive care, such as prophylactic antibiotics and immunoglobulin replacement therapy, and hematopoietic stem cell transplantation, which can provide a cure for the condition.

The discovery of Wiskott-Aldrich syndrome and subsequent research have contributed to a deeper understanding of the disorder, improved diagnostic capabilities, and potential avenues for therapeutic interventions. These advancements enhance the care and management of individuals affected by Wiskott-Aldrich syndrome.

What is Wiskott-Aldrich syndrome?

Wiskott-Aldrich syndrome (WAS) is a rare genetic disorder that affects the immune system and blood clotting. It is caused by mutations in the WAS gene, which codes for a protein called Wiskott-Aldrich protein (WASP). WASP is a protein that helps to control the development and function of white blood cells and platelets.

People with WAS have a decreased number of platelets, which are cells that help to clot blood. This can lead to easy bruising and bleeding. They also have a decreased number of white blood cells, which are cells that fight infection. This can make them more susceptible to infections.

WAS is inherited in an X-linked recessive manner. This means that the gene for WAS is located on the X chromosome, and males are more likely to be affected than females. Females who carry the gene for WAS are called carriers, but they usually do not have any symptoms.

There is no cure for WAS, but there are treatments that can help to manage the symptoms and improve quality of life. Treatment options may include:

Platelet transfusions: Platelet transfusions are used to treat bleeding.

Immunotherapy: Immunotherapy is a treatment that helps to boost the immune system. It may be used to treat infections or to prevent infections.

Bone marrow transplantation: Bone marrow transplantation is a procedure in which healthy bone marrow cells are transplanted into the body. This can be a cure for WAS, but it is a risky procedure.

The outlook for people with WAS varies depending on the severity of the disease. Some people with WAS live long and healthy lives, while others die in childhood.

If you or your child has been diagnosed with WAS, it is important to talk to your doctor about treatment options and how to best manage the disease. There are many resources available to help people with WAS and their families, such as the Wiskott-Aldrich Foundation and the National Organization for Rare Disorders (NORD).

Here are some additional information about WAS:

Symptoms: People with WAS may experience a variety of symptoms, including:

Easy bruising and bleeding

Frequent infections

Skin rashes

Eczema

Short stature

Immune thrombocytopenic purpura (ITP)

Leukemia

Diagnosis: WAS is diagnosed with a blood test that looks for decreased numbers of platelets and white blood cells. A genetic test can also be used to confirm the diagnosis.

Treatment: Treatment for WAS is aimed at managing the symptoms and preventing complications. Treatment options may include:

Platelet transfusions

Immunotherapy

Bone marrow transplantation

Prognosis: The prognosis for people with WAS varies depending on the severity of the disease. Some people with WAS live long and healthy lives, while others die in childhood.

Learn more about Wiskott-Aldrich syndrome from the Immune Deficiency Foundation

Immune Deficiency Foundation

7550 Teague Road, Suite 220

Hanover, MD 21076

Phone: 410-321-6647

Tell me about Diamond-Blackfan anemia

How was Diamond-Blackfan anemia discovered?

Diamond-Blackfan anemia (DBA) was discovered through the collaborative efforts of several researchers and clinicians. Here is an overview of how DBA was discovered:

Initial Observations: In 1938, two separate physicians, Dr. Louis Diamond in the United States and Dr. Kenneth Blackfan in Canada, independently described a group of children who presented with a profound form of anemia, macrocytosis (enlarged red blood cells), and physical abnormalities. They recognized the distinct clinical features of the condition and reported their findings.

Consolidation of Findings: In the 1960s, further research and case studies led to the consolidation of the clinical observations made by Diamond and Blackfan. The term "Diamond-Blackfan anemia" was coined to describe the disorder.

Genetic Link: In the 1980s, the genetic basis of Diamond-Blackfan anemia was discovered. Researchers identified mutations in genes involved in ribosome biogenesis and protein synthesis as the underlying cause of the condition. These genes include RPS19, RPS24, RPS17, and other ribosomal protein genes. Dysfunction of these genes affects the production of red blood cells in the bone marrow.

Identification of DBA-Associated Genes: Over the years, advances in genetic research and sequencing technologies have led to the identification of additional genes associated with DBA. Mutations in these genes disrupt various aspects of ribosome biogenesis and function, impairing red blood cell production.

Diagnostic Advances: The discovery of DBA-associated genes has facilitated the development of genetic testing methods for diagnosing Diamond-Blackfan anemia. Genetic testing can identify mutations in these genes, confirm the diagnosis, determine the subtype of DBA, and provide genetic counseling for affected families. Additionally, laboratory tests can assess red blood cell parameters and bone marrow function to support the diagnosis of DBA.

Research and Treatment: Ongoing research in Diamond-Blackfan anemia aims to deepen the understanding of the disease mechanisms, explore potential therapeutic strategies, and develop interventions that address the underlying genetic and cellular defects. Treatment options for DBA include blood transfusions to manage anemia, corticosteroids to stimulate red blood cell production, and, in some cases, stem cell transplantation.

The discovery of Diamond-Blackfan anemia and subsequent research have contributed to improved diagnostic methods, a better understanding of the disease's genetic basis and cellular mechanisms, and the development of interventions that enhance the care and management of individuals with Diamond-Blackfan anemia.

What is Diamond-Blackfan anemia?

Diamond-Blackfan anemia (DBA) is a rare, inherited blood disorder that affects the bone marrow. It is characterized by a decrease in the production of red blood cells, which carry oxygen to the body's tissues. This can lead to a variety of health problems, including anemia, fatigue, shortness of breath, and pale skin.

DBA is caused by mutations in one of several genes that are involved in the development of red blood cells. These mutations lead to a defect in the way that the bone marrow produces red blood cells.

DBA is inherited in an autosomal dominant manner, which means that only one mutated copy of the gene is needed for a person to develop the disease. However, not everyone who inherits a mutated gene will develop DBA. The risk of developing DBA is higher if the mutated gene is inherited from a parent who has the disease.

The symptoms of DBA can vary from person to person, but they typically begin in early childhood. Common symptoms include:

Anemia: Anemia is a condition in which the body does not have enough red blood cells. This can lead to fatigue, shortness of breath, and pale skin.

Short stature: People with DBA are often shorter than average.

Facial abnormalities: People with DBA may have facial abnormalities, such as a small jaw, high cheekbones, and a small nose.

Other symptoms: People with DBA may also experience other symptoms, such as:

Frequent infections

Heart problems

Kidney problems

Bone problems

Increased risk of cancer

There is no cure for DBA. Treatment is aimed at managing the symptoms and preventing complications. Treatment options may include:

Blood transfusions: Blood transfusions are used to treat anemia and to prevent complications, such as stroke and heart attack.

Growth hormone therapy: Growth hormone therapy can help to improve growth and development.

Bone marrow transplantation: Bone marrow transplantation is a procedure in which healthy bone marrow cells are transplanted into the body. This can be a cure for DBA, but it is a risky procedure.

The outlook for people with DBA varies depending on the severity of the disease. Some people with DBA live long and healthy lives, while others die in childhood.

If you or your child has been diagnosed with DBA, it is important to talk to your doctor about treatment options and how to best manage the disease. There are many resources available to help people with DBA and their families, such as the Diamond Blackfan Anemia Foundation and the National Organization for Rare Disorders (NORD).

Learn more about Diamond-Blackfan anema from the Diamond Blackfan Anemia Foundation, Inc.

Diamond Blackfan Anemia Foundation, Inc.

P.O. Box 1092

West Seneca, New York 14224

1-716-674-2818

Tell me about Severe combined immunodeficiency (SCID)

How was Severe combined immunodeficiency (SCID) discovered?

Severe combined immunodeficiency (SCID) was discovered through the collaborative efforts of several researchers and clinicians. Here is an overview of how SCID was discovered:

Early Observations: In the mid-20th century, clinicians observed a group of children who displayed severe and recurrent infections, failure to thrive, and a lack of immune responses to infections and vaccines. These observations suggested a profound deficiency in immune system function.

Bubble Boy: In the 1970s and 1980s, the case of a young boy named David Vetter, often referred to as the "Bubble Boy," brought significant attention to SCID. David Vetter lived in a sterile plastic bubble to protect him from infections due to his compromised immune system. His case highlighted the devastating consequences of SCID and the urgent need for further research and understanding.

Identification of Genetic Basis: In the 1990s, breakthrough discoveries identified the genetic basis of SCID. Researchers found that mutations in various genes involved in immune system development and function could lead to SCID. These genes include those encoding cytokine receptors, enzymes involved in DNA repair, and components of the immune system signaling pathways.

X-Linked SCID: One of the most well-known forms of SCID is X-linked SCID, which primarily affects boys. In 1993, researchers identified that mutations in the common gamma chain (γc) gene, which is shared by several cytokine receptors, were responsible for X-linked SCID. This discovery shed light on the critical role of the γc cytokine receptor in immune cell development and function.

Other Forms of SCID: Subsequent research identified various other genetic mutations associated with different forms of SCID, including ADA deficiency SCID, JAK3 deficiency SCID, and RAG deficiency SCID, among others. Each subtype of SCID is characterized by distinct genetic abnormalities affecting different components of the immune system.

Diagnostic Advances: The discovery of specific genetic mutations associated with SCID has significantly improved diagnostic capabilities. Genetic testing can now identify these mutations, confirm the diagnosis of SCID, determine the subtype of SCID, and provide genetic counseling for affected families. Additionally, immunological and functional assays can assess immune cell populations and function to support the diagnosis of SCID.

Treatment Options: SCID is a life-threatening condition, and early detection is crucial. Treatment options for SCID include hematopoietic stem cell transplantation, gene therapy, and enzyme replacement therapy, depending on the specific subtype and available interventions.

The discovery of SCID and subsequent research have led to significant advancements in understanding the genetic basis of the condition, improved diagnostic methods, and the development of targeted treatments. These advancements have contributed to improved outcomes and quality of life for individuals with SCID.

What is Severe combined immunodeficiency (SCID) ?

Severe combined immunodeficiency (SCID) is a rare, life-threatening genetic disorder that affects the immune system. People with SCID have a severely weakened immune system that makes them very susceptible to infections.

SCID is caused by mutations in genes that are involved in the development of T cells and B cells, which are two types of white blood cells that play important roles in the immune system. Without T cells and B cells, people with SCID are unable to fight off infections, which can lead to serious and life-threatening complications.

There are different types of SCID, each caused by a different mutation in a different gene. The most common type of SCID is adenosine deaminase (ADA) deficiency, which is caused by a mutation in the ADA gene. ADA is an enzyme that helps to break down a waste product called adenosine. When ADA is deficient, adenosine builds up in the body and can damage T cells and B cells.

SCID is usually diagnosed in early childhood. Symptoms of SCID can include:

- Frequent infections, such as pneumonia, meningitis, and sepsis
- Failure to thrive

- Slow growth
- Recurrent diarrhea
- Skin infections
- Mouth sores
- Easy bruising
- Bleeding

If you or your child is experiencing any of these symptoms, it is important to see a doctor right away. SCID is a serious condition, but it can be treated with early diagnosis and treatment.

There are two main treatments for SCID: bone marrow transplantation and gene therapy. Bone marrow transplantation is a procedure in which healthy bone marrow cells are transplanted into the body. This can replace the damaged T cells and B cells and restore the immune system. Gene therapy is a treatment that involves changing the DNA of cells to correct the mutation that causes SCID. This is a newer treatment, but it has shown promise in some cases.

With early diagnosis and treatment, people with SCID can live long and healthy lives.

Learn more about Severe combined immunodeficiency from IDF

Immune Deficiency Foundation

7550 Teague Road, Suite 220

Hanover, Maryland 21076

Tell me about Chronic granulomatous disease (CGD)

How was Chronic granulomatous disease (CGD) discovered?

Chronic granulomatous disease (CGD) was discovered through the collaborative efforts of several researchers and clinicians. Here is an overview of how CGD was discovered:

Observations of Clinical Features: In the mid-20th century, clinicians noticed a group of patients who presented with recurrent and severe bacterial and fungal infections, particularly involving certain organs and tissues, such as the lungs, skin, and lymph nodes. These infections were characterized by the formation of granulomas, which are clusters of immune cells.

Discovery of an Immunodeficiency: In 1954, a group of researchers led by Dr. Jan J. C. Snapper described a patient who displayed a specific pattern of recurrent infections, including pneumonia and abscesses. They recognized that the patient had a defect in the function of phagocytes, a type of immune cell responsible for engulfing and destroying pathogens. This defect in phagocyte function was identified as an underlying immunodeficiency, which later became known as chronic granulomatous disease.

Abnormal Oxidative Burst: Subsequent studies in the 1960s and 1970s by Dr. John L. Fahey and others revealed that individuals with CGD had impaired ability of phagocytes to generate reactive oxygen species (ROS) through a process called the oxidative burst. This impaired oxidative burst led to the inability to effectively kill certain types of bacteria and fungi, making individuals with CGD highly susceptible to these infections.

Identification of Genetic Basis: In the 1980s and 1990s, researchers made significant progress in identifying the genetic basis of CGD. They discovered that mutations in genes encoding subunits of the NADPH oxidase enzyme complex, which is responsible for generating ROS in phagocytes, were responsible for CGD. These genes include CYBB, CYBA, NCF1, NCF2, and NCF4, among others.

Diagnostic Advances: The identification of genetic mutations associated with CGD has greatly improved diagnostic capabilities. Genetic testing can now identify these mutations, confirm the diagnosis of CGD, determine the specific subtype of CGD, and provide genetic counseling for affected families. Additionally, functional assays can assess the oxidative burst capacity of phagocytes to support the diagnosis of CGD.

Treatment Options: Currently, there is no cure for CGD, but various treatment options are available to manage the condition. These include prophylactic antibiotic therapy, antifungal medications, immunoglobulin replacement therapy, and hematopoietic stem cell transplantation. In recent years, gene therapy approaches have also shown promise in treating certain forms of CGD.

The discovery of CGD and subsequent research have deepened our understanding of the genetic and immunological basis of the disease, improved diagnostic methods, and led to the development of treatment strategies that can help individuals with CGD lead healthier lives.

What is Chronic granulomatous disease (CGD) ?

Chronic granulomatous disease (CGD) is a rare, inherited disorder that affects the body's ability to fight infections. People with CGD have a defect in a gene that controls the production of an enzyme called NADPH oxidase. NADPH oxidase is important for the production of reactive oxygen species (ROS), which are chemicals that help to kill bacteria and other harmful organisms.

Without ROS, people with CGD are unable to fight off infections effectively. This can lead to a variety of infections, including pneumonia, meningitis, and abscesses. People with CGD are also at increased risk of developing certain types of cancer, such as lymphoma and leukemia.

CGD is inherited in an autosomal recessive manner, which means that both parents must carry a mutated copy of the gene in order for their child to be born with the disease.

There is no cure for CGD, but there are treatments that can help to prevent and treat infections. Treatment options may include:

Antibiotics: Antibiotics are used to treat infections.

G-CSF: Granulocyte colony-stimulating factor (G-CSF) is a medication that helps to increase the number of white blood cells in the body.

Bone marrow transplantation: Bone marrow transplantation is a procedure in which healthy bone marrow cells are transplanted into the body. This can be a cure for CGD, but it is a risky procedure.

With early diagnosis and treatment, people with CGD can live long and healthy lives.

Here are some additional information about CGD:

Symptoms: People with CGD may experience a variety of symptoms, including:

Frequent infections, such as pneumonia, meningitis, and abscesses

Failure to thrive

Slow growth

Recurrent diarrhea

Skin infections

Mouth sores

Easy bruising

Bleeding

Diagnosis: CGD is diagnosed with a blood test that looks for decreased numbers of neutrophils and increased numbers of immature white blood cells. A genetic test can also be used to confirm the diagnosis.

Treatment: Treatment for CGD is aimed at preventing and treating infections. Treatment options may include:

Antibiotics

G-CSF

Bone marrow transplantation

Prognosis: The prognosis for people with CGD varies depending on the severity of the disease. Some people with CGD live long and healthy lives, while others die in childhood.

Learn more about Chronic granulomatous disease from the CGD Society

CGD Society

PO Box 454

Dartford DA1 9PE

0800 987 8988

Tell me about Hyper-IgE syndrome

How was Hyper-IgM syndrome discovered?

Hyper-IgM syndrome (HIGM) was discovered through the collaborative efforts of several researchers and clinicians. Here is an overview of how HIGM was discovered:

Observation of Immunodeficiency: In the mid-1960s, clinicians observed a group of patients who displayed recurrent and severe infections, particularly involving the respiratory and gastrointestinal tracts. These patients had normal or elevated levels of immunoglobulin M (IgM), but significantly reduced levels of other types of immunoglobulins, such as IgG, IgA, and IgE.

Recognition of a Distinct Syndrome: Based on these clinical observations, it was recognized that these patients had a distinct immunodeficiency syndrome characterized by elevated IgM levels and deficiency of other immunoglobulin isotypes. This condition was later named Hyper-IgM syndrome.

Identification of Genetic Basis: In the late 1990s and early 2000s, the genetic basis of Hyper-IgM syndrome was discovered. Researchers identified that mutations in specific genes involved in the class-switching process of B cells were responsible for different subtypes of HIGM. The most common form of HIGM, known as HIGM1, is caused by mutations in the CD40 ligand (CD40L) gene, while other forms, such as HIGM2 and HIGM3, are caused by mutations in the AICDA and CD40 genes, respectively.

Defective T-Cell Signaling: The discovery of CD40L mutations in HIGM1 led to the understanding that this protein plays a crucial role in the interaction between T cells and B cells. CD40L on activated T cells interacts with CD40 on B cells, triggering signals necessary for B cell class-switching and production of different immunoglobulin isotypes. Defects in CD40L disrupt this interaction, leading to the hyperproduction of IgM and deficiency of other immunoglobulins.

Clinical and Laboratory Advances: The identification of genetic mutations associated with HIGM has facilitated improved diagnostic capabilities. Genetic testing can now identify these mutations, confirm the diagnosis of HIGM, determine the specific subtype of HIGM, and provide genetic counseling for affected families. Additionally, laboratory tests can assess the levels of immunoglobulins and evaluate T-cell function to support the diagnosis of HIGM.

Treatment Options: Management of HIGM typically involves immunoglobulin replacement therapy to provide the deficient immunoglobulin isotypes, prophylactic antibiotics to prevent infections, and other supportive measures. Hematopoietic stem cell transplantation may be considered for severe cases or when a suitable donor is available.

The discovery of Hyper-IgM syndrome and subsequent research have deepened our understanding of the genetic and immunological basis of the disease, improved diagnostic methods, and informed the development of treatment strategies that can help individuals with HIGM live healthier lives.

What is Hyper-IgM syndrome?

Hyper-IgM syndrome (HIGM) is a rare, inherited immunodeficiency disorder characterized by recurrent infections and low levels of immunoglobulins (Igs) other than IgM. Igs are proteins produced by the immune system that help fight infection.

There are three types of HIGM, each caused by a different genetic defect. The most common type is X-linked HIGM, which is caused by a mutation in the CD40 ligand gene. The other two types are autosomal recessive HIGM1 and autosomal recessive HIGM2, which are caused by mutations in the CD40 gene and the activation-induced cytidine deaminase (AID) gene, respectively.

People with HIGM are susceptible to a variety of infections, including pneumonia, meningitis, sepsis, and infections of the skin, ears, and sinuses. They are also at increased risk of developing autoimmune disorders, such as rheumatoid arthritis and lupus.

There is no cure for HIGM, but there are treatments that can help prevent and treat infections. Treatment options may include:

Antibiotics: Antibiotics are used to treat infections.

Immunoglobulin therapy: Immunoglobulin therapy involves injecting the patient with antibodies from healthy donors. This can help to boost the immune system and fight off infections.

Bone marrow transplantation: Bone marrow transplantation is a procedure in which healthy bone marrow cells are transplanted into the body. This can be a cure for HIGM, but it is a risky procedure.

With early diagnosis and treatment, people with HIGM can live long and healthy lives.

Here are some additional information about HIGM:

Symptoms: People with HIGM may experience a variety of symptoms, including:

Frequent infections, such as pneumonia, meningitis, and sepsis

Failure to thrive

Slow growth

Recurrent diarrhea

Skin infections

Mouth sores

Easy bruising

Bleeding

Diagnosis: HIGM is diagnosed with a blood test that looks for low levels of IgG, IgA, and IgE, and normal or elevated levels of IgM. A genetic test can also be used to confirm the diagnosis.

Treatment: Treatment for HIGM is aimed at preventing and treating infections. Treatment options may include:

Antibiotics

Immunoglobulin therapy

Bone marrow transplantation

Prognosis: The prognosis for people with HIGM varies depending on the severity of the disease. Some people with HIGM live long and healthy lives, while others die in childhood.

Learn more about Hyper-IgM syndrome from the HyperIgM Foundation

Hyper IgM Foundation

680 W END AVE, APT 12D

New York, NY 10025

Tell me about Myelodysplastic syndromes (MDS)

How was Myelodysplastic syndromes (MDS) discovered?

Myelodysplastic syndromes (MDS) are a group of disorders characterized by abnormal production of blood cells in the bone marrow. The discovery and understanding of MDS involved a series of scientific observations and advancements. Here is an overview of the historical developments in the discovery of MDS:

Early Observations: In the early 20th century, clinicians and pathologists observed a group of patients who presented with symptoms of anemia, bleeding, and increased susceptibility to infections. These patients had abnormal bone marrow findings, including dysplastic (abnormal) cells and ineffective blood cell production. However, at that time, the condition was not clearly differentiated as a distinct entity.

Recognition as a Syndrome: In the 1950s and 1960s, hematologists began recognizing that certain patients had a common set of features, including cytopenias (low blood cell counts), dysplastic bone marrow changes, and an increased risk of progression to acute leukemia. This led to the recognition of a distinct clinical syndrome, which was later termed "myelodysplastic syndrome" or MDS.

Classification Systems: Over the years, researchers developed classification systems to categorize and subclassify MDS based on various factors, such as the percentage of abnormal cells in the bone marrow, the types of blood cells affected, and the presence of specific genetic abnormalities. These classification systems, such as the French-American-British (FAB) classification and the World Health Organization (WHO) classification, provide guidelines for diagnosing and classifying different types and subtypes of MDS.

Advancements in Cytogenetics and Molecular Studies: With advancements in cytogenetic and molecular techniques, researchers discovered specific genetic abnormalities and chromosomal alterations associated with MDS. For example, the identification of certain chromosomal abnormalities, such as deletions or rearrangements of genetic material, provided important insights into the underlying genetic changes driving MDS development and progression.

Risk Stratification and Treatment Advances: Researchers developed risk stratification systems based on various clinical, cytogenetic, and molecular factors to predict the prognosis and guide treatment decisions for individuals with MDS. Different risk categories help tailor therapy accordingly. Treatment approaches for MDS include supportive care, blood transfusions, growth factors, immunosuppressive therapy, and in some cases, hematopoietic stem cell transplantation.

Continued Research: Ongoing research in MDS focuses on understanding the molecular and cellular mechanisms involved in the development and progression of the disease. Scientists are investigating novel targeted therapies, immunotherapies, and epigenetic modulators to improve treatment outcomes. Clinical trials and collaborative efforts are also essential in advancing our knowledge and finding new therapeutic strategies.

The discovery and ongoing research in MDS have significantly contributed to improved diagnostic techniques, better risk stratification, and the development of tailored treatment options, leading to improved outcomes and quality of life for individuals affected by this group of disorders.

What is Myelodysplastic syndromes (MDS)?

Myelodysplastic syndromes (MDS) are a group of bone marrow disorders that affect the production of blood cells. In MDS, the bone marrow makes too few healthy blood cells or makes abnormal blood cells that do not work properly. This can lead to a number of problems, including anemia, infection, and bleeding.

MDS is a relatively rare disease, affecting about 15,000 people in the United States each year. The average age of diagnosis is 65, but MDS can occur at any age.

The cause of MDS is unknown, but it is thought to be caused by a combination of genetic and environmental factors. Some factors that may increase the risk of developing MDS include:

Age: The risk of developing MDS increases with age.

Exposure to radiation: Exposure to radiation, such as from ionizing radiation or from certain medical treatments, can increase the risk of developing MDS.

Exposure to certain chemicals: Exposure to certain chemicals, such as benzene, can increase the risk of developing MDS.

Certain genetic conditions: Certain genetic conditions, such as Down syndrome, can increase the risk of developing MDS.

Previous chemotherapy or radiation treatment: People who have been treated with chemotherapy or radiation therapy for other cancers are at an increased risk of developing MDS.

The symptoms of MDS can vary from person to person. Common symptoms include:

Fatigue: Feeling tired or weak all the time

Pale skin: Pale skin due to anemia

Easy bruising: Bruising easily due to low platelet counts

Frequent infections: Frequent infections due to low white blood cell counts

Bone pain: Bone pain due to the cancer cells in the bone marrow

Swollen lymph nodes: Swollen lymph nodes in the neck, underarms, or groin

Night sweats: Night sweats that are profuse enough to soak the bedclothes

Unexplained weight loss: Unexplained weight loss

If you experience any of these symptoms, it is important to see a doctor for diagnosis and treatment. Early diagnosis and treatment can improve the chances of a cure.

The treatment for MDS depends on the type of MDS, the stage of the disease, and the patient's overall health. Treatment options may include:

Observation: In some cases, MDS may be mild enough that no treatment is needed. The doctor will monitor the patient closely to see if the disease progresses.

Chemotherapy: Chemotherapy uses drugs to kill cancer cells. Chemotherapy is often used to treat MDS that is more advanced.

Stem cell transplantation: Stem cell transplantation is a procedure in which healthy stem cells are transplanted into the patient's body to replace the stem cells that have been damaged by MDS. Stem cell transplantation is often used to treat MDS that is very advanced or that has not responded to other treatments.

The outlook for people with MDS varies depending on the type of MDS, the stage of the disease, and the patient's overall health. The median survival time for people with MDS is about 3 years. However, some people with MDS live for many years without any problems.

Learn more about Myelodysplastic syndromes from the MDS Foundation

The MDS Foundation

4573 South Broad St., Suite 150

Yardville, NJ 08620

1-(800)-637-0839

Outside the US only:

1-609-298-1035

Tell me about Acute myeloid leukemia (AML)

How was Acute myeloid leukemia (AML) discovered?

The discovery and understanding of acute myeloid leukemia (AML), a type of cancer that affects the bone marrow and blood, involved a series of scientific observations and advancements. Here is an overview of the historical developments in the discovery of AML:

Early Observations: In the 19th century, physicians and pathologists noted the presence of abnormal cells in the bone marrow and blood of individuals with acute leukemia. However, at that time, leukemia was not differentiated into specific subtypes.

Differentiation from Acute Lymphoblastic Leukemia: In the mid-20th century, researchers recognized that leukemia could be classified into different subtypes based on the type of cells involved. The distinction between acute lymphoblastic leukemia (ALL) and acute myeloid leukemia (AML) was made through microscopic examination and immunophenotyping techniques. AML was characterized by the presence of abnormal myeloid cells, a type of immature white blood cell, in the bone marrow and blood.

Morphological Classification: Pathologists played a crucial role in defining and classifying AML based on the appearance of the leukemia cells. They identified various subtypes of AML, such as promyelocytic leukemia (APL), myelomonocytic leukemia, and monocytic leukemia, among others. These subtypes were characterized by distinct morphological features observed under the microscope.

Cytogenetic and Molecular Studies: Advances in cytogenetic and molecular techniques further contributed to the understanding of AML. Researchers discovered specific chromosomal abnormalities and genetic mutations associated with different AML subtypes. For example, the identification of the Philadelphia chromosome, a genetic abnormality involving the fusion of two genes, helped differentiate a subset of AML called Philadelphia chromosome-positive AML.

Improved Diagnostic Techniques: Over time, advancements in diagnostic techniques, such as flow cytometry and molecular testing, have enhanced the accuracy and speed of AML diagnosis. These techniques allow for the identification of specific cell surface markers and genetic abnormalities associated with AML, aiding in subtype classification and treatment planning.

Risk Stratification and Treatment Advances: Researchers developed risk stratification systems based on various clinical, cytogenetic, and molecular factors to guide treatment decisions for individuals with AML. Different subtypes of AML may respond differently to treatment, so risk stratification helps tailor therapy accordingly. Treatment approaches have evolved to include chemotherapy regimens, targeted therapies, and stem cell transplantation, leading to improved outcomes for certain AML subtypes.

Continued Research: Ongoing research in AML focuses on understanding the underlying biology of the disease, identifying novel genetic mutations, exploring targeted therapies, and developing more effective treatment strategies. Clinical trials and collaborative efforts contribute to advancements in treatment options and the quest for improved outcomes for patients with AML.

The discovery and ongoing research in AML have significantly contributed to improved diagnostic techniques, better risk stratification, and the development of tailored treatment options, leading to improved survival rates and quality of life for individuals affected by this type of leukemia.

What is Acute myeloid leukemia (AML)?

Acute myeloid leukemia (AML) is a type of cancer that starts in the bone marrow. The bone marrow is where blood cells are made. In AML, the bone marrow makes too many immature white blood cells called myeloid cells. These myeloid cells are called blasts. Blasts do not work properly and cannot fight infection. They can also crowd out healthy blood cells, which can lead to problems such as anemia, infection, and bleeding.

The risk of developing AML increases with age. The average age of diagnosis is 66. Other factors that may increase the risk of developing AML include:

Exposure to radiation: Exposure to radiation, such as from ionizing radiation or from certain medical treatments, can increase the risk of developing AML.

Exposure to certain chemicals: Exposure to certain chemicals, such as benzene, can increase the risk of developing AML.

Certain genetic conditions: Certain genetic conditions, such as Down syndrome, can increase the risk of developing AML.

Previous chemotherapy or radiation treatment: People who have been treated with chemotherapy or radiation therapy for other cancers are at an increased risk of developing AML.

The symptoms of AML can vary from person to person. Common symptoms include:

Fatigue: Feeling tired or weak all the time

Pale skin: Pale skin due to anemia

Easy bruising: Bruising easily due to low platelet counts

Frequent infections: Frequent infections due to low white blood cell counts

Bone pain: Bone pain due to the cancer cells in the bone marrow

Swollen lymph nodes: Swollen lymph nodes in the neck, underarms, or groin

Night sweats: Night sweats that are profuse enough to soak the bedclothes

Unexplained weight loss: Unexplained weight loss

If you experience any of these symptoms, it is important to see a doctor for diagnosis and treatment. Early diagnosis and treatment can improve the chances of a cure.

The treatment for AML usually involves a combination of chemotherapy and radiation therapy. Chemotherapy uses drugs to kill cancer cells. Radiation therapy uses high-energy beams to kill cancer cells.

The type of treatment that is best for you will depend on the stage of your cancer and your overall health.

The outlook for people with AML has improved significantly in recent years. The cure rate for AML is now about 60% for people under the age of 65 and about 35% for people over the age of 65. The outlook is even better for people who are diagnosed and treated early.

Here are some things you can do to reduce your risk of developing AML:

Get regular checkups: It is important to see your doctor for regular checkups, even if you feel healthy. This will allow your doctor to detect any problems early, when they are easier to treat.

Avoid smoking: Smoking increases your risk of developing cancer.

Limit alcohol intake: Excessive alcohol intake increases your risk of developing cancer.

Get vaccinated: There are vaccines that can help to protect you from some types of cancer.

Learn more about Acute myeloid leukemia from the <u>Leukemia & Lymphoma Society</u>

The Leukemia & Lymphoma Society

3 International Drive, Suite 200

Rye Brook, NY 10573

(888) 557-7177

Tell me about Acute lymphoblastic leukemia (ALL)

How was Acute lymphoblastic leukemia (ALL) discovered?

Acute lymphoblastic leukemia (ALL), a type of cancer that affects the white blood cells, was discovered and characterized through a series of scientific advancements and observations. Here is an overview of the historical developments in the discovery of ALL:

Early Observations: In the late 19th century, pathologists noted the presence of abnormal cells in the bone marrow and blood of individuals with acute leukemia. However, at that time, leukemia was not differentiated into specific subtypes.

Differentiation from Acute Myeloid Leukemia: In the mid-20th century, researchers recognized that leukemia could be divided into different subtypes based on the type of cells involved. The distinction between acute lymphoblastic leukemia (ALL) and acute myeloid leukemia (AML) was made through microscopic examination and immunophenotyping techniques. ALL was characterized by the presence of abnormal lymphoblasts, a type of immature white blood cell, in the bone marrow and blood.

Advancements in Immunophenotyping: In the 1970s and 1980s, the development of immunophenotyping techniques revolutionized the identification and classification of leukemia. By using antibodies that could recognize and bind to specific proteins on the surface of cells, researchers were able to differentiate between different subtypes of leukemia, including ALL. Immunophenotyping allowed for more accurate diagnosis and classification of ALL based on the specific markers expressed on the lymphoblasts.

Cytogenetic and Molecular Studies: As technology advanced, cytogenetic and molecular studies became instrumental in understanding the genetic and molecular abnormalities associated with ALL. Researchers discovered specific chromosomal alterations and genetic mutations that play a role in the development and progression of the disease. For example, the identification of the Philadelphia chromosome, a genetic abnormality involving the fusion of two genes, helped differentiate a subset of ALL called Philadelphia chromosome-positive ALL.

Risk Stratification and Treatment Advances: Over time, researchers developed risk stratification systems based on various clinical and genetic factors to guide treatment decisions for individuals with ALL. This allowed for more personalized and targeted therapies, resulting in improved outcomes. Chemotherapy protocols were refined, and additional treatment modalities, such as hematopoietic stem cell transplantation and targeted therapies, were introduced to further enhance the management of ALL.

Continued Research: Ongoing research in ALL aims to deepen our understanding of the disease's biology, identify new genetic and molecular abnormalities, explore novel treatment approaches, and improve long-term outcomes for patients. Clinical trials and collaborative efforts contribute to advancements in treatment strategies and the development of more effective therapies.

The discovery and ongoing research in ALL have significantly contributed to improved diagnostic techniques, better risk stratification, and the development of tailored treatment options, leading to improved survival rates and quality of life for individuals affected by this type of leukemia.

What is Acute lymphoblastic leukemia (ALL)?

Acute lymphoblastic leukemia (ALL) is a type of cancer that starts in the bone marrow. The bone marrow is where blood cells are made. In ALL, the bone marrow makes too many immature white blood cells called lymphocytes. These lymphocytes are called lymphoblasts. Lymphoblasts do not work properly and cannot fight infection. They can also crowd out healthy blood cells, which can lead to problems such as anemia, infection, and bleeding.

ALL is the most common type of cancer in children. It is also the most common type of leukemia in adults under the age of 25. The risk of developing ALL increases with age.

The cause of ALL is unknown. However, there are some factors that may increase the risk of developing ALL, such as:

Exposure to radiation: Exposure to radiation, such as from ionizing radiation or from certain medical treatments, can increase the risk of developing ALL.

Exposure to certain chemicals: Exposure to certain chemicals, such as benzene, can increase the risk of developing ALL.

Certain genetic conditions: Certain genetic conditions, such as Down syndrome, can increase the risk of developing ALL.

The symptoms of ALL can vary from person to person. Common symptoms include:

Fatigue: Feeling tired or weak all the time

Pale skin: Pale skin due to anemia

Easy bruising: Bruising easily due to low platelet counts

Frequent infections: Frequent infections due to low white blood cell counts

Bone pain: Bone pain due to the cancer cells in the bone marrow

Swollen lymph nodes: Swollen lymph nodes in the neck, underarms, or groin

Night sweats: Night sweats that are profuse enough to soak the bedclothes

Unexplained weight loss: Unexplained weight loss

If you experience any of these symptoms, it is important to see a doctor for diagnosis and treatment. Early diagnosis and treatment can improve the chances of a cure.

The treatment for ALL usually involves a combination of chemotherapy and radiation therapy. Chemotherapy uses drugs to kill cancer cells. Radiation therapy uses high-energy beams to kill cancer cells.

The type of treatment that is best for you will depend on the stage of your cancer and your overall health.

The outlook for people with ALL has improved significantly in recent years. The cure rate for ALL is now about 85% for children and about 65% for adults. The outlook is even better for people who are diagnosed and treated early.

Here are some things you can do to reduce your risk of developing ALL:

Get regular checkups: It is important to see your doctor for regular checkups, even if you feel healthy. This will allow your doctor to detect any problems early, when they are easier to treat.

Avoid smoking: Smoking increases your risk of developing cancer.

Limit alcohol intake: Excessive alcohol intake increases your risk of developing cancer.

Get vaccinated: There are vaccines that can help to protect you from some types of cancer.

Learn more about Acute lymphoblastic leukemia from St. Jude Children's Research Hospital

St. Jude Children's Research Hospital

262 Danny Thomas Place

Memphis, TN 38105

866 2785 5833

Tell me about Non-Hodgkin lymphoma (NHL)

How was Non-Hodgkin lymphoma (NHL) discovered?

Non-Hodgkin lymphoma (NHL) is a diverse group of cancers that affect the lymphatic system. The discovery and understanding of NHL as a distinct entity separate from Hodgkin lymphoma involved contributions from several researchers and advancements in medical knowledge. Here is an overview of the historical developments in the discovery of NHL:

Differentiation from Hodgkin Lymphoma: The recognition of NHL as a distinct disease entity from Hodgkin lymphoma began in the mid-20th century. As medical knowledge advanced, researchers and pathologists noted differences in the clinical features, microscopic appearance, and behavior of certain lymphomas that did not fit the characteristics of Hodgkin lymphoma.

Revised Classification Systems: In the late 20th century, several classification systems were developed to better categorize and subdivide NHL based on various factors, including cell type, growth pattern, and clinical behavior. The Revised European-American Lymphoma (REAL) classification and later the World Health Organization (WHO) classification systems provided standardized guidelines for diagnosing and classifying different types of NHL.

Advancements in Technology: The development of advanced diagnostic techniques, particularly immunohistochemistry and molecular genetic studies, has significantly contributed to the understanding of NHL. These techniques allow for more accurate identification of specific cell types and genetic abnormalities associated with different subtypes of NHL.

Identification of Subtypes: Through research and the application of molecular techniques, scientists have identified various subtypes of NHL, each with its unique clinical, pathological, and genetic features. These subtypes include diffuse large B-cell lymphoma (DLBCL), follicular lymphoma, mantle cell lymphoma, marginal zone lymphoma, and many others.

Genetic and Molecular Insights: Further studies have revealed specific genetic alterations and molecular mechanisms involved in the development and progression of NHL. These insights have led to a better understanding of the disease's underlying biology and have opened doors for targeted therapies and personalized treatment approaches.

Improved Treatment Strategies: Over time, advances in chemotherapy, immunotherapy, and targeted therapies have revolutionized the treatment of NHL. Researchers have developed more effective and less toxic treatment regimens, leading to improved outcomes and survival rates for patients with NHL.

Ongoing Research: Research in NHL continues to expand our knowledge of the disease. Scientists are investigating new therapeutic targets, studying mechanisms of drug resistance, exploring immunotherapy approaches, and developing novel treatment strategies.

It's important to note that NHL encompasses a wide range of subtypes, each with its unique characteristics and clinical behavior. As research progresses, a deeper understanding of NHL subtypes and their respective treatment options will continue to evolve, ultimately leading to improved outcomes for patients affected by this group of cancers.

What is Non-Hodgkin lymphoma (NHL)?

Non-Hodgkin lymphoma (NHL) is a type of cancer that starts in the lymphocytes, a type of white blood cell. Lymphocytes are part of the immune system, which helps the body fight infection. In NHL, the lymphocytes grow out of control and form tumors in the lymph nodes.

There are many different types of NHL, and they are classified according to how the cancer cells look under a microscope. The most common type of NHL is diffuse large B-cell lymphoma.

NHL is more common in older adults, but it can occur at any age. The risk of developing NHL increases with age, exposure to certain chemicals, and certain genetic conditions.

The symptoms of NHL can vary from person to person. Common symptoms include:

Enlarged lymph nodes: The most common symptom of NHL is enlarged lymph nodes. These nodes are often painless and can be found in the neck, underarms, or groin.

Fever: People with NHL may experience fevers that are not caused by an infection.

Night sweats: People with NHL may experience night sweats that are profuse enough to soak their bedclothes.

Unexplained weight loss: People with NHL may lose weight without trying to.

Chest pain: People with NHL may experience chest pain, which can be caused by a tumor pressing on the heart or lungs.

Other symptoms: People with NHL may experience other symptoms, such as fatigue, shortness of breath, itching, and fatigue.

If you experience any of these symptoms, it is important to see a doctor for diagnosis and treatment. Early diagnosis and treatment can improve the chances of a cure.

The treatment for NHL depends on the type of NHL, the stage of the cancer, and the patient's overall health. Treatment options may include:

Chemotherapy: Chemotherapy uses drugs to kill cancer cells.

Radiation therapy: Radiation therapy uses high-energy beams to kill cancer cells.

Stem cell transplantation: Stem cell transplantation is a procedure in which healthy stem cells are transplanted into the patient's body to replace the stem cells that have been damaged by chemotherapy or radiation therapy.

Targeted therapy: Targeted therapy uses drugs that target specific molecules on cancer cells.

Immunotherapy: Immunotherapy uses the body's own immune system to fight cancer.

The outlook for people with NHL varies depending on the type of NHL, the stage of the cancer, and the patient's overall health. The cure rate for NHL is about 70%. The outlook is even better for people who are diagnosed and treated early.

Here are some things you can do to reduce your risk of developing NHL:

Get regular checkups: It is important to see your doctor for regular checkups, even if you feel healthy. This will allow your doctor to detect any problems early, when they are easier to treat.

Eat a healthy diet: A healthy diet can help to boost your immune system and reduce your risk of developing cancer.

Exercise regularly: Exercise can help to boost your immune system and reduce your risk of developing cancer.

Avoid smoking: Smoking increases your risk of developing cancer.

Limit alcohol intake: Excessive alcohol intake increases your risk of developing cancer.

Get vaccinated: There are vaccines that can help to protect you from some types of cancer.

Learn more about Non-Hodgkin lymphoma from the <u>Lymphoma Research Foundation</u>

The Lymphoma Research Foundation

Wall Street Plaza

88 Pine Street, Suite 2400

New York, NY 10005

212-349-2910

800-500-9976

Tell me about Hodgkin lymphoma?

How was Hodgkin lymphoma discovered?

Hodgkin lymphoma was first described and identified by Dr. Thomas Hodgkin, an English physician, in the early 19th century. Dr. Hodgkin made groundbreaking observations and published a series of papers detailing his findings on a distinct type of lymphatic cancer.

In 1832, Dr. Hodgkin presented a lecture at the Medical and Chirurgical Society of London where he described several cases of patients with a particular form of lymphadenopathy (enlarged lymph nodes). He noted that these patients exhibited common clinical features, such as painless swelling of lymph nodes, systemic symptoms, and characteristic microscopic features upon examination of affected tissues.

Dr. Hodgkin's meticulous anatomical and pathological investigations allowed him to differentiate this specific form of lymphadenopathy from other diseases presenting with similar symptoms. He described the unique characteristics of the cancer cells and their distribution within the lymph nodes, highlighting the disease's distinct nature.

Following his initial publication, Dr. Hodgkin continued to document and study cases, refining his observations and further characterizing the disease. The term "Hodgkin's disease" was eventually coined to recognize his significant contributions to its identification and understanding.

Over time, advancements in medical knowledge and technology have led to a deeper understanding of Hodgkin lymphoma. Researchers have discovered specific subtypes of the disease, identified genetic and molecular alterations, and developed more refined diagnostic and staging criteria.

Importantly, the introduction of effective treatments, such as combination chemotherapy and radiation therapy, has significantly improved the prognosis and survival rates for individuals with Hodgkin lymphoma.

Continued research efforts are focused on unraveling the underlying mechanisms, further refining diagnostic techniques, exploring targeted therapies, and improving the overall management of Hodgkin lymphoma. Through ongoing scientific investigation, we strive to

enhance our understanding of the disease and develop more personalized and effective treatment approaches.

What is Hodgkin lymphoma?

Hodgkin lymphoma is a type of cancer that affects the lymphatic system. The lymphatic system is part of the immune system and helps to fight infection. In Hodgkin lymphoma, abnormal white blood cells called Reed-Sternberg cells grow out of control and form tumors in the lymph nodes.

Hodgkin lymphoma is a relatively rare cancer, accounting for about 1% of all cancers. It is most common in people between the ages of 15 and 35, and again after the age of 55.

The cause of Hodgkin lymphoma is unknown, but it is thought to be caused by a combination of genetic and environmental factors. There is no known way to prevent Hodgkin lymphoma.

The symptoms of Hodgkin lymphoma can vary from person to person. Common symptoms include:

- Enlarged lymph nodes: The most common symptom of Hodgkin lymphoma is enlarged lymph nodes. These nodes are often painless and can be found in the neck, underarms, or groin.

- Fever: People with Hodgkin lymphoma may experience fevers that are not caused by an infection.

- Night sweats: People with Hodgkin lymphoma may experience night sweats that are profuse enough to soak their bedclothes.

- Unexplained weight loss: People with Hodgkin lymphoma may lose weight without trying to.

- Chest pain: People with Hodgkin lymphoma may experience chest pain, which can be caused by a tumor pressing on the heart or lungs.

- Other symptoms: People with Hodgkin lymphoma may experience other symptoms, such as fatigue, shortness of breath, itching, and fatigue.

If you experience any of these symptoms, it is important to see a doctor for diagnosis and treatment. Early diagnosis and treatment can improve the chances of a cure.

Treatment for Hodgkin lymphoma usually involves a combination of chemotherapy and radiation therapy. Chemotherapy uses drugs to kill cancer cells. Radiation therapy uses high-energy beams to kill cancer cells.

The type of treatment that is best for you will depend on the stage of your cancer and your overall health.

The outlook for people with Hodgkin lymphoma is good. The cure rate for Hodgkin lymphoma is about 85%. The outlook is even better for people who are diagnosed and treated early.

Here are some things you can do to reduce your risk of developing Hodgkin lymphoma:

- Get regular checkups: It is important to see your doctor for regular checkups, even if you feel healthy. This will allow your doctor to detect any problems early, when they are easier to treat.

- Eat a healthy diet: A healthy diet can help to boost your immune system and reduce your risk of developing cancer.

- Exercise regularly: Exercise can help to boost your immune system and reduce your risk of developing cancer.

- Avoid smoking: Smoking increases your risk of developing cancer.

- Limit alcohol intake: Excessive alcohol intake increases your risk of developing cancer.

- Get vaccinated: There are vaccines that can help to protect you from some types of cancer.

Learn more about Hodgkin lymphoma from Lymphoma action

Tell me about Multiple sclerosis (MS)

How was Multiple sclerosis (MS) discovered?

The discovery and understanding of multiple sclerosis (MS) involved contributions from several physicians and researchers over the course of history. Here is an overview of the historical developments in the discovery of MS:

Jean-Martin Charcot: The French neurologist Jean-Martin Charcot played a significant role in the early recognition and description of multiple sclerosis. In the late 19th century, Charcot provided detailed clinical observations and conducted autopsies on individuals with MS. He described the characteristic symptoms and physical findings, including the presence of lesions in the central nervous system.

Early Descriptions: Before Charcot, there were scattered reports of individuals with symptoms similar to MS. Scottish physician Robert Carswell, in 1838, described the microscopic appearance of MS lesions in the brain and spinal cord. English physician Sir Augustus d'Esté Courtenay also made similar observations in 1849.

Discovery of Demyelination: In the early 20th century, researchers recognized that MS is characterized by demyelination, which is the destruction of the protective myelin sheath surrounding nerve fibers in the central nervous system. Demyelination leads to disruptions in nerve signaling and the characteristic symptoms seen in MS.

Diagnostic Criteria: In 1965, an international panel of experts established the Schumacher criteria, which provided standardized guidelines for the diagnosis of MS. Over time, these criteria have been revised and updated to improve the accuracy and consistency of MS diagnosis.

Advancements in Imaging: The development of imaging techniques, particularly magnetic resonance imaging (MRI), revolutionized the diagnosis and monitoring of MS. In the 1980s, MRI scans became an essential tool for visualizing MS lesions in the brain and spinal cord, allowing for earlier and more accurate detection of the disease.

Immunological Insights: Research in the latter half of the 20th century focused on the immune system's role in MS. It was discovered that MS is an autoimmune disease, where the

body's immune system mistakenly attacks the myelin sheath. This immune-mediated damage contributes to the development and progression of MS.

Genetic and Environmental Factors: Studies have indicated that both genetic and environmental factors contribute to the risk of developing MS. Certain genetic variations have been associated with an increased susceptibility to the disease, while environmental factors, such as vitamin D levels, infections, and geographical location, have been linked to disease prevalence.

Ongoing Research: MS research continues to advance our understanding of the disease. Scientists are investigating potential triggers, studying the mechanisms of immune system dysfunction, exploring neuroprotective strategies, and developing new treatments aimed at reducing inflammation and promoting myelin repair.

While significant progress has been made in understanding MS, there is still much to learn about the disease's complex nature. Continued research efforts hold the promise of further unraveling the underlying mechanisms and improving the diagnosis, treatment, and management of MS.

What is Multiple sclerosis (MS)?

Multiple sclerosis (MS) is a chronic disease that affects the central nervous system (CNS). The CNS is made up of the brain, spinal cord, and optic nerves. In MS, the immune system attacks the myelin sheath, a protective layer that surrounds nerve fibers. This damage can slow down or block messages traveling between the brain and the rest of the body.

MS is a lifelong disease, but it is not always disabling. Some people with MS have mild symptoms that do not interfere with their daily lives. Others may have more severe symptoms that can make it difficult to walk, work, or care for themselves.

The symptoms of MS can vary from person to person and can change over time. Common symptoms include:

Fatigue: Feeling tired or weak all the time

Vision problems: Blurry vision, double vision, or loss of vision

Numbness or tingling: Tingling or numbness in the hands, arms, legs, or face

Weakness: Muscle weakness in the arms, legs, or trunk

Slurred speech: Difficulty speaking or understanding speech

Trouble walking: Difficulty walking, balance problems, or falls

Bladder or bowel problems: Difficulty controlling the bladder or bowels

Heat sensitivity: Worsening of symptoms with heat

The cause of MS is unknown, but it is thought to be caused by a combination of genetic and environmental factors. There is no cure for MS, but there are treatments that can help to manage the symptoms and slow the progression of the disease. Treatment for MS may include:

Medication: There are a number of medications that can help to manage the symptoms of MS. These medications work by suppressing the immune system and preventing further damage to the myelin sheath.

Physical therapy: Physical therapy can help to maintain muscle strength and range of motion.

Occupational therapy: Occupational therapy can help with activities of daily living, such as dressing, bathing, and eating.

Support groups: Support groups can provide emotional support and information to people with MS and their families.

If you think you may have MS, it's important to see a doctor for diagnosis and treatment. Early diagnosis and treatment can help to improve quality of life and slow the progression of the disease.

Learn more about Multiple Sclerosis from the National Multiple Sclerosis Society

1-800-344-4867

Tell me about Amyotrophic lateral sclerosis (ALS)

How was Amyotrophic lateral sclerosis (ALS) discovered?

Amyotrophic lateral sclerosis (ALS), also known as Lou Gehrig's disease, was first identified and described by several physicians in the 19th century. The discovery and understanding of ALS involved contributions from multiple researchers over time. Here is an overview of the historical developments in the discovery of ALS:

Jean-Martin Charcot: The renowned French neurologist Jean-Martin Charcot made significant contributions to the understanding of ALS in the late 19th century. Charcot's detailed clinical observations and studies on patients with ALS helped establish it as a distinct neurological disorder. He described the characteristic symptoms of muscle weakness, spasticity, and muscle wasting, and emphasized the involvement of both upper and lower motor neurons.

Naming of ALS: The term "amyotrophic lateral sclerosis" was coined by Pierre Marie, a French neurologist and student of Charcot, in 1889. "Amyotrophic" refers to the muscle atrophy (wasting) seen in the disease, "lateral" indicates the involvement of the lateral corticospinal tracts in the spinal cord, and "sclerosis" refers to the hardening and scarring of these tracts.

El Escorial Criteria: In the 20th century, the El Escorial criteria were established to provide standardized diagnostic criteria for ALS. These criteria, developed in the 1990s, outline specific clinical and electrophysiological features necessary for a definitive diagnosis of ALS.

Discovery of Motor Neuron Degeneration: In the mid-20th century, researchers began to focus on understanding the underlying pathology of ALS. It was discovered that the disease primarily affects motor neurons, the nerve cells responsible for controlling voluntary muscle movement. Degeneration and death of these motor neurons lead to muscle weakness and eventual paralysis.

Role of Glutamate Excitotoxicity: Research in the 1990s highlighted the role of glutamate excitotoxicity in ALS. It was observed that excessive release of the neurotransmitter glutamate, coupled with impaired removal, leads to overstimulation of motor neurons and subsequent cell damage.

Genetic Discoveries: In the past few decades, significant progress has been made in identifying genetic factors associated with ALS. The discovery of mutations in the superoxide dismutase 1 (SOD1) gene in some familial cases of ALS in 1993 was a breakthrough. Since then, other genes, including C9orf72, TARDBP, FUS, and others, have been linked to familial and sporadic forms of the disease.

Advancements in Research: Ongoing research continues to explore the complex mechanisms involved in ALS, including oxidative stress, protein misfolding, mitochondrial dysfunction, and immune system involvement. Animal models, cell-based studies, and advancements in genetic analysis techniques have contributed to a deeper understanding of ALS pathogenesis.

While significant progress has been made in understanding ALS, there is still much to learn about the disease. Research efforts continue to focus on identifying potential therapeutic targets, developing new treatment strategies, and improving the care and quality of life for individuals affected by ALS.

What is Amyotrophic lateral sclerosis (ALS) ?

Amyotrophic lateral sclerosis (ALS), also known as Lou Gehrig's disease, is a progressive neurodegenerative disease that affects nerve cells in the brain and spinal cord. These nerve cells control voluntary muscle movement, and when they die, the muscles weaken and waste away.

ALS is a fatal disease, and there is no cure. However, there are treatments that can help to slow the progression of the disease and improve quality of life.

The most common symptoms of ALS include:

Weakness: Muscles become weak and tire easily.

Spasticity: Muscles become stiff and difficult to move.

Fasciculations: Involuntary muscle twitching.

Speech problems: Difficulty speaking, swallowing, and chewing.

Breathing problems: Difficulty breathing, especially at night.

ALS is a rare disease, affecting about 1 in 30,000 people. The average age of onset is 55, but it can occur at any age.

The cause of ALS is unknown, but it is thought to be caused by a combination of genetic and environmental factors. There is no known way to prevent ALS.

Treatment for ALS focuses on managing the symptoms and improving quality of life. There is no cure for ALS, but there are treatments that can help to slow the progression of the disease and improve quality of life. These treatments include:

Medication: There are a number of medications that can help to manage the symptoms of ALS. These medications work by improving muscle strength, reducing spasticity, and improving speech and swallowing.

Physical therapy: Physical therapy can help to maintain muscle strength and range of motion.

Speech therapy: Speech therapy can help to improve communication skills.

Occupational therapy: Occupational therapy can help with activities of daily living, such as dressing, bathing, and eating.

Palliative care: Palliative care is a type of care that focuses on relieving the symptoms and side effects of ALS. Palliative care can also help to improve quality of life for people with ALS and their families.

If you think you may have ALS, it's important to see a doctor for diagnosis and treatment. Early diagnosis and treatment can help to improve quality of life and slow the progression of the disease.

Learn more about Amyotrophic lateral sclerosis from the ALS Association

ALS Association National Office

1300 Wilson Boulevard, Suite 600

Arlington, VA 22209

(800) 782-4747

Tell me about Parkinson's disease

How was Parkinson's disease discovered?

Parkinson's disease was first identified and described by Dr. James Parkinson, a British physician, in 1817. Dr. Parkinson published a paper titled "An Essay on the Shaking Palsy," in which he detailed his observations of six individuals who exhibited similar symptoms.

In his essay, Dr. Parkinson described the main features of the condition, which included resting tremors, rigidity, bradykinesia (slowness of movement), and postural instability. He noted that these symptoms were associated with a progressive degenerative process affecting the nervous system.

Dr. Parkinson's work was significant because it was the first systematic description of what would later be recognized as Parkinson's disease. He provided a clinical picture of the condition and distinguished it from other movement disorders of the time.

Over the years, further research and scientific advancements have expanded our understanding of Parkinson's disease. In the 1960s, the discovery of a connection between dopamine deficiency and Parkinson's symptoms led to the development of levodopa, a medication that became a cornerstone of Parkinson's treatment.

Subsequent studies identified the loss of dopamine-producing cells in a region of the brain called the substantia nigra as a central feature of Parkinson's disease. The accumulation of abnormal protein deposits called Lewy bodies in brain cells is also recognized as a characteristic pathological feature of the disease.

Advancements in brain imaging techniques, such as positron emission tomography (PET) and magnetic resonance imaging (MRI), have enabled researchers to visualize the changes that occur in the brains of individuals with Parkinson's disease. This has provided further insights into the underlying mechanisms and progression of the disease.

While the exact cause of Parkinson's disease remains unknown, research suggests a combination of genetic and environmental factors play a role. Ongoing research focuses on understanding the disease's mechanisms, developing new treatment strategies, and

exploring potential neuroprotective approaches to slow or halt the progression of Parkinson's.

The discovery and ongoing research surrounding Parkinson's disease have greatly advanced our knowledge of the condition, leading to improved diagnosis, treatment options, and a better understanding of the impact it has on individuals and their families.

What is Parkinson's disease?

Parkinson's disease (PD) is a progressive neurological disorder that affects movement. It's caused by the loss of nerve cells in the brain that produce a chemical called dopamine. Dopamine helps control movement, and when it's not produced in sufficient amounts, it can cause a variety of symptoms, including tremors, slowness of movement, stiffness, and impaired balance and coordination.

Parkinson's disease is not contagious and is not a result of lifestyle choices. It's thought to be caused by a combination of genetic and environmental factors. There is no cure for Parkinson's disease, but there are treatments that can help to manage the symptoms and improve quality of life.

The most common symptoms of Parkinson's disease include:

- Tremors: These are involuntary, rhythmic movements that usually affect the hands, arms, legs, and face.
- Slowness of movement: This is called bradykinesia. People with Parkinson's disease may have difficulty starting or stopping movements, and they may walk with a shuffling gait.
- Stiffness: This is called rigidity. People with Parkinson's disease may have difficulty moving their limbs because their muscles are stiff.
- Impaired balance and coordination: This can lead to falls.
- Other symptoms: People with Parkinson's disease may also experience other symptoms, such as fatigue, depression, anxiety, and sleep problems.

Parkinson's disease is a progressive disease, which means that the symptoms get worse over time. The rate at which the disease progresses varies from person to person. Some people with Parkinson's disease can live relatively normal lives for many years, while others may need more help as the disease progresses.

There is no cure for Parkinson's disease, but there are treatments that can help to manage the symptoms and improve quality of life. The most common treatments for Parkinson's disease are:

- Medication: There are a number of medications that can help to improve the symptoms of Parkinson's disease. These medications work by increasing the levels of dopamine in the brain.

- Surgery: In some cases, surgery may be an option for people with Parkinson's disease. Surgery can help to improve the symptoms of tremors and movement problems.

- Physical therapy: Physical therapy can help to improve balance, coordination, and range of motion.

- Speech therapy: Speech therapy can help to improve communication skills.

- Occupational therapy: Occupational therapy can help with activities of daily living, such as dressing, bathing, and eating.

- Support groups: Support groups can provide emotional support and information to people with Parkinson's disease and their families.

If you think you may have Parkinson's disease, it's important to see a doctor for diagnosis and treatment. Early diagnosis and treatment can help to improve quality of life and slow the progression of the disease.

Learn more about Parkinson's disease from the Parkinson's Foundation

Parkinson's Foundation
200 SE 1st Street, Ste 800

Miami, FL 33131, USA

Parkinson's Foundation

1359 Broadway, Ste 1509

New York, NY 10018, USA

Tell me about Alzheimer's disease

How was Alzheimer's disease discovered?

Alzheimer's disease was first discovered and described by Dr. Alois Alzheimer, a German psychiatrist and neuropathologist, in 1906. Dr. Alzheimer made this groundbreaking discovery while working with a patient named Auguste Deter.

Auguste Deter, a middle-aged woman, was experiencing memory loss, language difficulties, and behavioral changes. Her condition progressively worsened, leading to severe cognitive decline. After her death, Dr. Alzheimer had the opportunity to examine her brain during an autopsy.

During the examination, Dr. Alzheimer observed significant abnormalities in the brain tissue, including the presence of plaques and tangles. Plaques are clumps of a protein called beta-amyloid that accumulate between nerve cells, while tangles are twisted fibers of a protein called tau that accumulate inside nerve cells.

These distinctive brain abnormalities, which Dr. Alzheimer referred to as "senile plaques" and "neurofibrillary tangles," became the hallmarks of the disease he described. Dr. Alzheimer recognized that these pathological changes in the brain were responsible for the neurological symptoms exhibited by Auguste Deter during her life.

Dr. Alzheimer presented his findings in a lecture in 1906 and published a detailed case study on Auguste Deter's condition. His work laid the foundation for the understanding of what would later be known as Alzheimer's disease.

Since Dr. Alzheimer's initial discovery, extensive research has been conducted to further understand the causes, risk factors, progression, and treatment options for Alzheimer's disease. The identification of genetic mutations associated with familial forms of Alzheimer's disease and advancements in brain imaging techniques have contributed to our current understanding of the disease.

Alzheimer's disease is now recognized as the most common form of dementia, a progressive neurological disorder that affects memory, thinking, behavior, and the ability to perform daily activities. Ongoing research continues to focus on finding better diagnostic tools,

understanding the underlying mechanisms, and developing potential treatments to improve the lives of individuals affected by Alzheimer's disease.

What is Alzheimer's disease?

Alzheimer's disease is a progressive brain disorder that causes memory loss and other cognitive decline. It is the most common cause of dementia, a general term for loss of memory and other cognitive abilities severe enough to interfere with daily life.

Alzheimer's disease is not a normal part of aging. The risk of developing Alzheimer's disease increases with age, but it can occur at any age.

The exact cause of Alzheimer's disease is unknown, but it is believed to be caused by a combination of genetic and environmental factors.

The symptoms of Alzheimer's disease can vary from person to person, but they often include:

- Memory loss: This is the most common symptom of Alzheimer's disease. People with Alzheimer's disease may forget recent events, names, and faces.

- Confusion: People with Alzheimer's disease may become confused about time, place, and people.

- Personality changes: People with Alzheimer's disease may become withdrawn, irritable, or aggressive.

- Trouble thinking and problem-solving: People with Alzheimer's disease may have difficulty with simple tasks, such as paying bills or cooking a meal.

- Changes in language: People with Alzheimer's disease may have difficulty finding the right words or understanding what others are saying.

- Vision and spatial problems: People with Alzheimer's disease may have difficulty seeing or judging distances.

There is no cure for Alzheimer's disease, but there are treatments that can help to slow the progression of the disease and manage the symptoms. Treatment for Alzheimer's disease may include:

- Medications: There are a number of medications that can help to slow the progression of Alzheimer's disease. These medications work by increasing the levels of acetylcholine, a neurotransmitter that is important for memory and thinking.

- Non-medication treatments: There are a number of non-medication treatments that can help to manage the symptoms of Alzheimer's disease. These treatments include:

    o Memory training: Memory training exercises can help to improve memory and cognitive function.

    o Social activities: Social activities can help to reduce stress and improve mood.

    o Physical activity: Physical activity can help to improve overall health and well-being.

    o Diet: A healthy diet can help to improve cognitive function and reduce the risk of developing Alzheimer's disease.

There are a number of things that you can do to reduce your risk of developing Alzheimer's disease, including:

- Eat a healthy diet: A healthy diet can help to improve cognitive function and reduce the risk of developing Alzheimer's disease.

- Exercise regularly: Physical activity can help to improve overall health and well-being.

- Stay mentally active: Mental activities, such as reading, playing games, and learning new things, can help to keep your brain healthy.

- Get enough sleep: Sleep is important for memory and cognitive function.

- Manage stress: Stress can contribute to the development of Alzheimer's disease. Find healthy ways to manage stress, such as exercise, relaxation techniques, or spending time with loved ones.

- Don't smoke: Smoking can increase your risk of developing Alzheimer's disease.

- Limit alcohol intake: Excessive alcohol intake can increase your risk of developing Alzheimer's disease.

- Get regular checkups: If you have any concerns about your memory or thinking, see your doctor. Early diagnosis and treatment can help to slow the progression of Alzheimer's disease and improve quality of life.

Learn more about Alzheimer's disease from the Alzheimer's Association

Alzheimer's Association

225 N. Michigan Ave. Floor 17

Chicago, IL 60601

Tell me about Epilepsy

How was Epilepsy discovered?

Epilepsy is one of the oldest recorded neurological disorders, and its existence has been recognized for thousands of years. The understanding and recognition of epilepsy have evolved over time through observations and medical advancements. Here is a brief overview of the historical discovery and understanding of epilepsy:

Ancient Times: Epileptic seizures were described in ancient civilizations such as Mesopotamia, Egypt, and Greece. The ancient Greeks believed that seizures were caused by supernatural forces or gods and attributed them to divine intervention.

Hippocratic Era: The Greek physician Hippocrates (460-370 BCE), often regarded as the father of medicine, rejected the supernatural explanations of epilepsy and proposed that it had a natural origin in the brain. He believed that seizures were caused by an excess of black bile, one of the four bodily humors. This theory laid the foundation for the understanding of epilepsy as a medical condition.

Renaissance and Enlightenment: During the Renaissance, the supernatural beliefs surrounding epilepsy started to wane, and scholars began to search for physiological explanations. In the 17th and 18th centuries, researchers such as Thomas Willis and Jean-Baptiste Morgagni made significant contributions to the understanding of epilepsy as a neurological disorder.

Electroencephalography (EEG): The discovery of the electroencephalogram (EEG) in the early 20th century revolutionized the study of epilepsy. In 1924, Hans Berger, a German psychiatrist, recorded the electrical activity of the brain using electrodes placed on the scalp. This technique allowed the detection of abnormal electrical discharges during seizures, providing objective evidence of epilepsy.

Advancements in Treatment: The development of antiepileptic drugs (AEDs) in the mid-20th century greatly improved the management of epilepsy. The discovery of phenytoin in 1938 marked the beginning of modern AEDs. Since then, numerous medications have been developed to control seizures and improve the quality of life for people with epilepsy.

Research and Contemporary Understanding: In recent years, advancements in neuroscience and medical imaging techniques have deepened our understanding of epilepsy. Researchers have identified various causes of epilepsy, including genetic factors, brain injuries, infections, tumors, and developmental disorders. Advanced imaging technologies, such as magnetic resonance imaging (MRI) and positron emission tomography (PET), have helped in identifying structural and functional abnormalities in the brains of individuals with epilepsy.

It's important to note that epilepsy is a complex disorder with different types of seizures and causes, and ongoing research continues to expand our knowledge of this condition. While much progress has been made in the understanding and treatment of epilepsy, it remains an area of active investigation and medical research.

What is Epilepsy?

Epilepsy is a neurological disorder that causes recurrent seizures. A seizure is a sudden burst of electrical activity in the brain that can cause a variety of symptoms, including convulsions, loss of consciousness, and strange sensations or behavior.

Epilepsy is a common disorder, affecting about 1 in 26 people worldwide. It can occur at any age, but it is most common in children and adults under the age of 25.

There are many different types of epilepsy, and the cause of the disorder can vary from person to person. Some common causes of epilepsy include:

Brain injury: This can be caused by a traumatic brain injury, such as a car accident or a fall, or by a stroke.

Brain tumors: These can cause seizures by pressing on or damaging the brain tissue.

Genetic disorders: Some genetic disorders, such as Down syndrome and Angelman syndrome, are associated with an increased risk of epilepsy.

Infections: Some infections, such as meningitis and encephalitis, can damage the brain and lead to epilepsy.

Unknown causes: In about half of all cases, the cause of epilepsy is unknown.

Epilepsy is not contagious. It is also not a sign of mental illness.

The symptoms of a seizure can vary depending on the type of seizure. Some common symptoms include:

Convulsions: These are involuntary muscle contractions that can cause the person to fall to the ground.

Loss of consciousness: The person may lose consciousness for a few seconds or minutes.

Strange sensations or behavior: The person may experience strange sensations, such as a feeling of déjà vu or jamais vu, or they may behave in a way that is out of character for them.

After a seizure, the person may feel tired or confused. They may also have a headache or muscle pain.

Epilepsy is a lifelong condition, but it can be managed with medication. Most people with epilepsy can live normal, productive lives.

If you or someone you know has had a seizure, it is important to see a doctor. The doctor will perform a physical exam and may order tests, such as an EEG (electroencephalogram) or an MRI (magnetic resonance imaging), to diagnose the type of epilepsy and to rule out other possible causes of the seizures.

Once the type of epilepsy is diagnosed, the doctor can recommend a treatment plan. The most common treatment for epilepsy is medication. There are many different types of anti-epileptic drugs (AEDs), and the doctor will work with you to find the right medication for you.

If medication is not effective in controlling the seizures, the doctor may recommend other treatments, such as surgery or vagus nerve stimulation (VNS).

Surgery is an option for people with focal epilepsy, which is a type of epilepsy that is caused by abnormal electrical activity in a specific area of the brain. VNS is a non-surgical treatment that involves implanting a small device in the chest that sends electrical impulses to the vagus nerve.

Epilepsy is a complex disorder, but there are many resources available to help people with epilepsy and their families. The Epilepsy Foundation is a great resource for information and support. You can also find information and support online at the Epilepsy Foundation website.

Learn more about Epilepsy from the <u>Epilepsy Foundation</u>

Epilepsy Foundation

3540 Crain Highway, Suite 675,

Bowie, MD 20716

1.800.332.1000

Tell me about Cerebral palsy

How was Cerebral palsy discovered?

Although the first record of a case of cerebral palsy (CP) can be dated back to 1650, the condition was not formally identified until the late 1800s. In 1843, Scottish surgeon James Little published a paper describing a group of children with similar motor impairments. He noted that the children had all been born prematurely and that many of them had difficulty walking and talking. Little named the condition "Little's Disease" after himself.

In the early 1900s, American physician William John Osler published a book on CP that helped to increase awareness of the condition. Osler described the different types of CP and their causes. He also advocated for early intervention services for children with CP.

In the mid-1900s, there was a significant increase in research on CP. This research led to a better understanding of the causes of CP and to the development of new treatments. Today, there is no cure for CP, but there are treatments that can help to improve the quality of life for people with the condition.

Here are some of the causes of cerebral palsy:

Brain injury during pregnancy or childbirth: This is the most common cause of CP. It can be caused by problems with the placenta, the umbilical cord, or the baby's brain.

Brain infections: These can include meningitis, encephalitis, and cytomegalovirus (CMV) infection.

Genetic disorders: These can include Down syndrome, Prader-Willi syndrome, and Angelman syndrome.

Premature birth: Babies who are born prematurely are at increased risk for CP.

Low birth weight: Babies who are born with low birth weight are also at increased risk for CP.

The symptoms of CP can vary widely from person to person. Some people with CP may have mild symptoms, while others may have severe symptoms. Common symptoms of CP include:

Motor problems: These can include difficulty walking, running, and using the hands.

Speech problems: These can include difficulty speaking, understanding speech, and swallowing.

Learning disabilities: These can include difficulty with reading, writing, and math.

Epilepsy: This is a condition that causes seizures.

Vision problems: These can include difficulty seeing, double vision, and nystagmus (rapid eye movement).

Hearing problems: These can include difficulty hearing, deafness, and tinnitus (ringing in the ears).

There is no cure for CP, but there are treatments that can help to improve the quality of life for people with the condition. Treatment for CP may include:

Physical therapy: This can help to improve muscle strength and coordination.

Occupational therapy: This can help to improve fine motor skills and daily living skills.

Speech therapy: This can help to improve communication skills.

Special education: This can help children with CP learn at their own pace.

Medications: These can be used to treat seizures, spasticity, and pain.

Surgery: This may be used to correct deformities or to improve function.

With early intervention and support, people with CP can live long and fulfilling lives. They can attend school, hold jobs, and participate in activities in their communities. They can also make significant contributions to their families and to society.

What is Cerebral palsy?

Cerebral palsy is a group of neurological disorders that affect movement, muscle tone, and posture. It is caused by damage to the developing brain, usually before or during birth, but sometimes in early childhood. The term "cerebral" refers to the brain, and "palsy" refers to a disorder of movement or posture.

The specific cause of cerebral palsy is not always known, but it can result from various factors, including prenatal brain abnormalities, genetic mutations, maternal infections, premature birth, oxygen deprivation, traumatic brain injury, or certain complications during labor and delivery. The brain damage disrupts the normal communication between the brain and the muscles, leading to difficulties with muscle control and coordination.

The signs and symptoms of cerebral palsy can vary widely among individuals and may include:

Impaired movement and coordination: People with cerebral palsy often have difficulty with fine motor skills, such as grasping objects, writing, or buttoning clothes. They may also have challenges with gross motor skills, such as walking, running, or maintaining balance.

Muscle stiffness or rigidity: Some individuals with cerebral palsy experience increased muscle tone, which can cause muscle stiffness or tightness. This may affect their ability to move freely and result in abnormal posture or movements.

Abnormal reflexes: Certain reflexes that are typically present in infants may persist or be exaggerated in individuals with cerebral palsy. These abnormal reflexes can interfere with normal movements.

Spasticity or involuntary movements: Spastic cerebral palsy is the most common type and is characterized by muscle stiffness and spasms. Some individuals may also have involuntary movements or uncontrollable shaking (athetosis) or slow, writhing movements (dyskinesia).

Balance and coordination issues: Difficulties with balance and coordination can make activities that require precise movements, such as walking, difficult for individuals with cerebral palsy.

Speech and communication challenges: Some individuals with cerebral palsy may have difficulties with speech and language. This can range from mild speech impairments to more severe communication challenges.

Intellectual disabilities: While cerebral palsy primarily affects movement and posture, some individuals may also have intellectual disabilities. However, many people with cerebral palsy have normal intelligence.

Other associated conditions: Individuals with cerebral palsy may have other health issues, such as seizures, vision or hearing impairments, learning disabilities, or behavioral and emotional challenges.

Cerebral palsy is a lifelong condition, but with appropriate interventions and support, individuals can lead fulfilling lives. Treatment focuses on managing symptoms, promoting mobility and independence, and addressing associated medical and developmental concerns. This may involve a multidisciplinary approach, including physical and occupational therapy, speech and language therapy, assistive devices, medications for spasticity or pain management, and supportive educational and social services.

Early intervention is crucial for maximizing outcomes, and ongoing care and support are essential to address the changing needs of individuals with cerebral palsy as they grow and develop.

Learn more about Cerebral palsy from UCP

United Cerebral Palsy

8401 OLD COURTHOUSE RD.

VIENNA, VA 22182

Tell me about Down syndrome

How was Down syndrome discovered?

Down syndrome was first described in 1866 by John Langdon Down, a British physician. He described a group of children with similar physical features, including short stature, upward slanting eyes, and a flat facial profile. Down named the condition "Mongolian idiocy" because he believed that the children had physical features that resembled those of people from Mongolia.

In 1959, Jérôme Lejeune, a French physician, discovered that Down syndrome is caused by an extra copy of chromosome 21. This discovery led to a better understanding of the condition and to the development of new treatments.

Down syndrome is a genetic disorder that occurs when a person has three copies of chromosome 21 instead of the usual two copies. This extra copy of chromosome 21 causes a variety of physical and intellectual disabilities.

People with Down syndrome typically have short stature, upward slanting eyes, a flat facial profile, and a small jaw. They may also have heart defects, hearing loss, and thyroid problems. Intellectual disability is common in Down syndrome, and people with the condition may have difficulty with learning, language, and social skills.

There is no cure for Down syndrome, but there are treatments that can help to improve the quality of life for people with the condition. Treatment may include early intervention services, special education, and medical care for any associated health problems.

With early intervention and support, people with Down syndrome can live long and fulfilling lives. They can attend school, hold jobs, and participate in activities in their communities. They can also make significant contributions to their families and to society.

Here are some additional information about Down syndrome:

It is the most common chromosomal disorder, affecting about 1 in 700 births.

The exact cause of Down syndrome is unknown, but it is thought to be caused by a random error during cell division during early development.

There is no cure for Down syndrome, but there are treatments that can help to improve the symptoms.

People with Down syndrome typically have normal intelligence, but they may have some learning disabilities.

People with Down syndrome can have a normal life expectancy, but they may be at increased risk for certain health problems, such as heart disease, leukemia, and Alzheimer's disease.

If you have any concerns about your child's development, please talk to your doctor.

What is Down syndrome?

Down syndrome, also known as trisomy 21, is a genetic disorder caused by the presence of an extra copy of chromosome 21. It is named after John Langdon Down, the British physician who first described the condition in 1866. Down syndrome is characterized by a distinct set of physical features, intellectual disabilities, and various health conditions.

Typically, individuals have 46 chromosomes in each cell, with 23 inherited from each parent. In the case of Down syndrome, there is an additional copy of chromosome 21, resulting in a total of 47 chromosomes. This extra genetic material affects the development and functioning of the body and brain.

The features and characteristics of Down syndrome can vary, but some common signs and symptoms include:

Intellectual disabilities: Individuals with Down syndrome often have mild to moderate intellectual disabilities. The level of cognitive impairment can vary, but most individuals can develop basic academic and life skills with appropriate support and interventions.

Physical features: People with Down syndrome may have distinctive physical characteristics, including a flat facial profile, upward slanting eyes, a small nose, a protruding tongue, small and low-set ears, a short neck, and a single deep crease across the palm of the hand (known as a simian crease). They may also have decreased muscle tone (hypotonia) and shorter stature.

Developmental delays: Children with Down syndrome typically have delays in their physical and cognitive development, such as delayed speech and language skills, motor skills, and social development. Early intervention and specialized therapies can help support their development.

Health conditions: Individuals with Down syndrome have an increased risk of certain health conditions, including congenital heart defects, hearing loss, vision problems, thyroid disorders, gastrointestinal issues, respiratory infections, and an increased susceptibility to certain infections. Regular medical check-ups and appropriate management are important for addressing these associated health concerns.

Personality and social strengths: Individuals with Down syndrome often have friendly and sociable personalities. They can form strong bonds with family and friends, and they may exhibit empathy, warmth, and a genuine interest in others.

It's important to note that every individual with Down syndrome is unique, and the range and severity of symptoms can vary widely. With advances in medical care, early interventions, inclusive education, and supportive environments, individuals with Down syndrome can lead fulfilling lives and make significant contributions to their communities.

The diagnosis of Down syndrome is usually confirmed through a chromosomal analysis called a karyotype, which examines the number and structure of chromosomes. Prenatal testing, such as amniocentesis or chorionic villus sampling, can also detect the presence of an extra chromosome 21 before birth.

Supportive care, early intervention programs, educational opportunities, and medical management are essential components of managing Down syndrome. With appropriate interventions and support, individuals with Down syndrome can thrive and reach their full potential.

Learn more about Down Syndrome from ndss

National Down Syndrome Society

1155 15th Street NW

Suite 540

Washington, DC 20005

Telephone: 800-221-4602

Tell me about Turner syndrome

How was Turner syndrome discovered?

Turner syndrome was discovered in 1938 by Dr. Henry Turner, an American endocrinologist. He was studying a group of seven girls who had similar physical features, including short stature, webbed neck, and underdeveloped ovaries. Dr. Turner found that all of the girls had one X chromosome and no Y chromosome. He named the condition "Turner syndrome" after himself.

Turner syndrome is a genetic disorder that occurs when a female is born with only one X chromosome. This can happen because of a random error during cell division, or it can be inherited from a parent.

Girls with Turner syndrome typically have short stature, webbed neck, and underdeveloped ovaries. They may also have heart defects, kidney problems, and hearing loss. Intellectual disability is not common in Turner syndrome, but some girls may have learning disabilities.

There is no cure for Turner syndrome, but there are treatments that can help to improve the symptoms. Treatment may include growth hormone therapy, hormone replacement therapy, and surgery to correct heart defects or kidney problems.

With early diagnosis and treatment, girls with Turner syndrome can live long and healthy lives. They may experience challenges, but they can also achieve their goals and live fulfilling lives.

Here are some additional information about Turner syndrome:

It is the most common chromosomal disorder in females, affecting about 1 in 2,500 girls.

The exact cause of Turner syndrome is unknown, but it is thought to be caused by a random error during cell division during early development.

There is no cure for Turner syndrome, but there are treatments that can help to improve the symptoms.

Girls with Turner syndrome typically have normal intelligence, but they may have learning disabilities.

Girls with Turner syndrome can have a normal life expectancy, but they may be at increased risk for certain health problems, such as heart disease, kidney disease, and diabetes.

If you have any concerns about your child's development, please talk to your doctor.

What is Turner syndrome?

Turner syndrome, also known as 45,X or Monosomy X, is a genetic disorder that affects females. It is named after Henry Turner, an endocrinologist who first described the syndrome in 1938. Turner syndrome is characterized by the complete or partial absence of one of the X chromosomes in females.

Typically, females have two X chromosomes (XX), but in Turner syndrome, one X chromosome is either completely missing or partially deleted or altered. The specific chromosomal abnormality can vary, but the most common form is known as monosomy X, where only one X chromosome is present.

The features and symptoms of Turner syndrome can vary widely among affected individuals, but some common characteristics include:

Short stature: Girls with Turner syndrome often have slow growth and may have a significantly shorter stature than their peers. Growth hormone therapy can be used to promote growth in some cases.

Gonadal dysgenesis: Turner syndrome can lead to underdeveloped or absent ovaries, resulting in infertility and lack of secondary sexual characteristics during puberty. Most affected girls do not undergo normal puberty without hormone replacement therapy.

Physical features: Girls with Turner syndrome may have certain physical features, such as a webbed neck, low-set ears, a broad chest with widely spaced nipples, drooping eyelids (ptosis), and a high-arched palate.

Lymphedema: Swelling of the hands and feet due to a buildup of fluid (lymphedema) can occur in some individuals with Turner syndrome.

Cardiovascular abnormalities: There is an increased risk of congenital heart defects and other heart and blood vessel abnormalities in individuals with Turner syndrome.

Kidney problems: Some individuals may have structural abnormalities in the kidneys or urinary system.

Hearing loss: Hearing problems, such as partial hearing loss or complete deafness, can occur in a small percentage of individuals with Turner syndrome.

Learning difficulties: Some girls with Turner syndrome may have specific learning disabilities or difficulties with spatial and mathematical concepts. However, intelligence can vary widely among affected individuals.

Turner syndrome occurs randomly, and the specific cause of the chromosomal abnormalities is not well understood. Diagnosis is typically made through a chromosomal analysis called a karyotype, which examines the number and structure of chromosomes.

Early intervention and comprehensive medical care can help manage the symptoms and complications associated with Turner syndrome. Treatment may include growth hormone therapy to improve height, estrogen replacement therapy to induce puberty and support reproductive health, and ongoing monitoring and management of potential medical issues related to the heart, kidneys, and other affected systems. Regular check-ups, educational support, and psychosocial care are also important aspects of managing Turner syndrome.

Learn more about Turner Syndrome from Turner Syndrome Society of the United States

Turner Syndrome Society of the United States

11250 West Rd, Suite G

Houston, TX 77065

1-800-365-9944